Evaluating HIV/AIDS
Treatment Programs:
Innovative Methods
and Findings

Evaluating HIV/AIDS Treatment Programs: Innovative Methods and Findings has been co-published simultaneously as *Drugs & Society*, Volume 16, Numbers 1/2 2000.

Evaluating HIV/AIDS Treatment Programs: Innovative Methods and Findings

G. J. Huba, PhD
Editor

Lisa A. Melchior, PhD
Vivian B. Brown, PhD
Trudy A. Larson, MD
A. T. Panter, PhD
Associate Editors

Evaluating HIV/AIDS Treatment Programs: Innovative Methods and Findings has been co-published simultaneously as *Drugs & Society*, Volume 16, Numbers 1/2 2000.

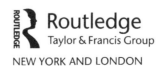

Routledge
Taylor & Francis Group

NEW YORK AND LONDON

First published 2000 by

The Haworth Press, Inc., 10 Alice Street, Binghamton, NY 13904-1580 USA

This edition published 2014 by Routledge
711 Third Avenue, New York, NY 10017, USA
2 Park Square, Milton Park, Abingdon, Oxon OX14 4RN

Routledge is an imprint of the Taylor & Francis Group, an informa business

Evaluating HIV/AIDS Treatment Programs: Innovative Methods and Findings has been co-published simultaneously as *Drugs & Society* ™ , Volume 16, Numbers 1/2 2000.

The development, preparation, and publication of this work has been undertaken with great care. However, the publisher, employees, editors, and agents of The Haworth Press and all imprints of The Haworth Press, Inc., including The Haworth Medical Press® and Pharmaceutical Products Press®, are not responsible for any errors contained herein or for consequences that may ensue from use of materials or information contained in this work. Opinions expressed by the author(s) are not necessarily those of The Haworth Press, Inc.

Cover design by Thomas J. Mayshock Jr.

Library of Congress Cataloging-in-Publication Data

Evaluating HIV/AIDS treatment programs : innovative methods and findings / G.J. Huba, editor ... [et al.].
   p. cm.
   "Co-published simultaneously as Drugs & Society, volume 16, number 1/2, 2000."
   Includes bibliographical references and index.
   ISBN 0-7890-1190-5 (alk. paper) – ISBN 0-7890-1191-3 (alk. paper)
   1. AIDS (Disease)–Patients–Care. 2. AIDS (Disease)–Patients–Services for. 3. Community health services. I. Huba, George J. II. Drugs & society.
RA644.A25 E924 2000
362.1'969792–dc21

                                            00-047218

Evaluating HIV/AIDS Treatment Programs: Innovative Methods and Findings

CONTENTS

ABOUT THE EDITORS

G. J. Huba, PhD, Editor, is President and Founder of The Measurement Group, a California-based consulting firm that specializes in social policy research, program evaluation, instrument development, and analysis. Dr. Huba was formerly on the faculties of UCLA and the University of Minnesota and Vice President of Research and Development at Western Psychological Services, a test publisher. A licensed psychologist, Dr. Huba received his PhD from Yale University in 1977. He is a fellow of the Evaluation, Measurement, and Statistics Division and the Addictions Division of the American Psychological Association. Dr. Huba is the author of more than 200 professional works in the technical areas of multivariate statistics, evaluation, the design of computerized expert systems and psychological instrumentation, innovative applications of the Internet for evaluation and information dissemination, and in the content areas of HIV services, substance abuse treatment and prevention, and large-scale human service delivery systems.

Lisa A. Melchior, PhD, Associate Editor, is Vice President of The Measurement Group, an applied social research and program evaluation firm. Prior to her work with The Measurement Group, Dr. Melchior coordinated projects in development at Western Psychological Services, a major publisher of psychological and educational tests. A licensed psychologist, Dr. Melchior received her PhD in psychological assessment from the University of Michigan in 1990. She is an active member of the American Psychological Association and the American Public Health Association. Dr. Melchior has published widely in the areas of survey research and evaluation of HIV/AIDS, substance abuse, and mental health services, particularly with respect to services for women and youth and persons with co-occurring disorders.

Vivian B. Brown, PhD, Associate Editor, is founder and Chief Executive Offier of PROTOTYPES, Centers for Innovation in Health, Mental Health and Social Services, a multi-facility, multi-service agency with services located throughout California and Washington, DC. Dr. Brown has more than 30 years of experience developing innovative, community-based services including Community Mental Health Centers and crisis intervention centers; residential, day treatment and outpatient drug abuse treatment services; HIV/AIDS outreach, prevention and interventions for women; specialized services for women, their children and their families;

mental health treatment and specialized dual diagnosis interventions; trauma and domestic violence prevention and intervention services. Dr. Brown received her PhD in Clinical Psychology from the University of Southern California. She is an adjunct Associate Professor of Psychiatry at UCLA and a fellow of the American Psychological Association. She is also a member of numerous federal, state, and local advisory committees and was elected as a Distinguished Practitioner in the National Academy of Practice Psychology.

Trudy A. Larson, MD, Associate Editor, is Professor of Pediatrics and Associate Dean of Primary Care Research, Education and Service at the University of Nevada School of Medicine. In this role she oversees all state and national outreach activities of the School of Medicine, including rural health system development, community-based medical education, public health program evaluation, continuing education for health professionals, health policy development, and the ongoing expansion and improvement of public health in Nevada through program innovation. Dr. Larson is the Medical Director of the Nevada Area AIDS Education and Training Center, the Principal Investigator of the Nevada AIDS Drug Assistance Program Comprehensive Evaluation Project, and a member of the Nevada State AIDS Advisory Board. A pediatric infectious disease specialist, she is the former Chair of the Department of Pediatrics at the University of Nevada School of Medicine where she has served since 1984.

A. T. Panter, PhD, Associate Editor (1989, New York University), is Associate Professor of Psychology in the L. L. Thurstone Psychometric Laboratory at the University of North Carolina, Chapel Hill. She is also a senior technical consultant at The Measurement Group. Dr. Panter's major research areas are measurement and test theory, multivariate data modeling, evaluation design, and individual differences. She has received several university-wide awards for her innovative approaches to teaching statistics and quantitative methodology to undergraduate and graduate students. Dr. Panter has been extensively involved in The Measurement Group's multi-site evaluation centers and has specialized in work with projects that provide technical assistance and/or health education/training to health care providers. She regularly consults with federal agencies on grant review, is a regular member of NIMH's grant panel on Risk, Prevention, and Health Behavior (RPHB-4), and serves on numerous national committees and editorial boards in the area of social/personality psychology and quantitative methods.

Foreword

It is well documented that substance use is a major factor in the current HIV/AIDS epidemic in the United States. Recent AIDS surveillance figures indicate that a minimum of 25% of new infections among males and 39% of new infections among females are directly associated with injecting drug use or with sex with a drug user (Centers for Disease Control and Prevention, 1999). These percents do not include the large numbers of individuals infected through sex with partners with unreported drug use, individuals with infections associated with non-injecting drug use, or those whose source of infection is unknown.

Men, women, and youth with HIV from all of these groups are described in the following Health Resources and Services Administration (HRSA) Special Projects of National Significance (SPNS) Cooperative Agreement papers. They come from very vulnerable populations who historically have not had access to ongoing health care. They may be homeless, lack health insurance, be discriminated against, and be diagnosed with additional co-morbidities. As the papers indicate, treating substance abuse and HIV involves service linkage and delivery that moves well beyond our traditional notions of medical care. It involves services that move from the treatment of addictions to linking HIV counseling and testing with early and ongoing treatment for both drug use and HIV, pre-release programs in correctional institutions with community care, and hepatitis C detection and HIV care.

To integrate such services, new program and policy models must be created. HRSA's SPNS Cooperative Agreement grantees have done this. The models and the evaluations that are presented here have implications not just for the approximately 2500 providers funded through the Ryan White CARE Act, but also for other community-based agencies and drug treatment programs that serve vulnerable populations.

As we search for improved ways of prolonging the lives of individuals

[Haworth co-indexing entry note]: "Foreword." O'Neill, Joseph F. and Katherine Marconi. Co-published simultaneously in *Drugs & Society* (The Haworth Press, Inc.) Vol. 16, No. 1/2, 2000, pp. xxi-xxii; and: *Evaluating HIV/AIDS Treatment Programs: Innovative Methods and Findings* (ed: G. J. Huba et al.) The Haworth Press, Inc., 2000, pp. xvii-xviii. Single or multiple copies of this article are available for a fee from The Haworth Document Delivery Service [1-800-342-9678, 9:00 a.m. - 5:00 p.m. (EST). E-mail address: getinfo@haworthpressinc.com].

xvii

diagnosed with HIV and for methods of successfully preventing new infections and co-morbid conditions from occurring, the SPNS models provide valuable lessons. The projects show that strong linkages can be established among community agencies with very different mandates, including substance abuse treatment, medical care, and correctional release case management. The successful project strategies tailor their interventions to their target populations–youth, women, immigrants, newly released inmates. And they point out very real issues, such as active client participation in treatment–issues that must be addressed. Most importantly, the information presented here on project clients and outcomes illustrates how community-based programs can be evaluated and best practices identified. Viewed as a whole, the Cooperative Agreement Projects indicate how Federal dollars can be invested in the development of new ways to deliver community health services.

Joseph F. O'Neill, MD, MPH
Associate Administrator
HIV/AIDS Bureau
HRSA

Katherine Marconi, PhD, MS
Director
Office of Science and Epidemiology
HIV/AIDS Bureau
HRSA

REFERENCE

Centers for Disease Control and Prevention. (1999). *HIV/AIDS Surveillance Report: U.S. HIV and AIDS cases reported through June 1999, 11*(1), 12.

Introduction

G. J. Huba, PhD
Lisa A. Melchior, PhD

In 1994, the U.S. Department of Health and Human Services (DHHS) Health Resources and Services Administration (HRSA), through its Special Projects of National Significance (SPNS) Program, funded 27 innovative models of HIV care. These projects, known collectively as the SPNS Cooperative Agreement, represented a diverse group of organizations with common goals–to improve access to care, health, and quality of life for traditionally underserved populations living with HIV/AIDS.

Indeed, the Cooperative Agreement Projects reached a high-need population. Enrollees across the various programs had the following characteristics: 6.0% were under age 21 or over age 55; 72.5% were people of color; 11.9% had a primary language other than English; 20.0% had children requiring care; 45.3% had less than 12 years of formal education; 85.7% were unemployed or not working; 88.9% were dependent on public support for medical insurance; 28.2% used or had used heroin; 44.9% used or had used crack cocaine; 56.9% used or had used another illicit drug; 54.2% had a current or prior alcohol problem; 49.7% were or had been involved with the criminal justice system; 22.1% engaged in current or prior sex work; 42.9% engaged in current or prior sex with an injection drug user; and 46.4% were without stable housing. The

---

G. J. Huba and Lisa A. Melchior are affiliated with The Measurement Group, Culver City, CA.

Address correspondence to: G. J. Huba, The Measurement Group, 5811A Uplander Way, Culver City, CA 90230 (E-mail: ghuba@TheMeasurementGroup.com).

This work was supported in part by the Health Resources and Services Administration (HRSA), HIV/AIDS Bureau (HAB), Special Projects of National Significance (SPNS) Grant No. 5 U90 HA 00030-05. This publication's contents are solely the responsibility of the authors and do not necessarily represent the official view of the funding agency.

[Haworth co-indexing entry note]: "Introduction" Huba, G. J., and Lisa A. Melchior. Co-published simultaneously in *Drugs & Society* (The Haworth Press, Inc.) Vol. 16, No. 1/2, 2000, pp. 1-3; and: *Evaluating HIV/AIDS Treatment Programs: Innovative Methods and Findings* (ed: G. J. Huba et al.) The Haworth Press, Inc., 2000, pp. 1-3. Single or multiple copies of this article are available for a fee from The Haworth Document Delivery Service [1-800-342-9678, 9:00 a.m. - 5:00 p.m. (EST). E-mail address: getinfo@haworthpressinc.com].

average number of these indices was 7.13 (standard deviation = 2.73, n = 1060) for males and 6.75 (standard deviation = 2.68, n = 1054) for females (t = 3.23 for the difference, degrees of freedom = 2112, $p < .001$). Almost all enrollees (87.7%) have four or more need-vulnerability factors (Huba, Melchior, Panter, and the HRSA/HAB SPNS Cooperative Agreement Steering Committee, 2000a).

This volume highlights the efforts of two clusters of projects within this initiative. One such group includes six programs identified as Community-Based Organizations (CBOs). The CBO projects share as a central theme the goal of providing high-quality care for individuals with HIV who belong to groups that are traditionally underserved because of linguistic, cultural, racial, and economic barriers that prevent their full integration into the traditional hospital-based service system. The other group featured here includes three projects that developed specialized medical care models within the context of a continuum of services in a medical clinic. These two groups of projects were included in this volume given that they collected similar data and shared a number of issues in evaluating their service models. A paper describing a study of end-stage AIDS care is also included as another example of applied research utilized by the Cooperative Agreement Projects. This volume also includes an overview of the HRSA HIV/AIDS Bureau (HAB) SPNS Cooperative Agreement grant initiative, a collaborative paper from each of the project work group clusters, and a paper detailing a number of conceptual issues in implementing program evaluation in these "real world" community organizations.

A growing resource for more information about these innovative HIV care models and their evaluations is available in an online Knowledge Base at www.TheMeasurementGroup.com. The Knowledge Base on Innovative Models of HIV/AIDS Care (Huba, Melchior, Panter, and the HRSA/HAB SPNS Cooperative Agreement Steering Committee, 2000b) presents pooled results from the Cooperative Agreement Projects and provides a method of rapid and wide information dissemination from this initiative via the Internet. The Knowledge Base builds on many of the results presented in this volume and is continuously updated and expanded. The Knowledge Base not only summarizes data from these projects in a highly accessible format, but also provides links to data collection forms and evaluation methods used to generate the information, as well as links to information about the service models that produced the featured results. We invite you to bookmark this resource and visit it often.

The work featured in this volume would not be possible without the contributions of a number of key individuals and organizations. First and foremost, funding from the Health Resources and Services Administration in the form of the cooperative agreements supported the efforts of the individual service models as well as the Evaluation and Dissemination Center that coordinated the multi-site evaluation. Throughout the five years of this initiative, Katherine Marconi, Ph.D., led the efforts in the HRSA Office of Science and Epidemiology. The SPNS Program itself was overseen initially by William Grace, Ph.D., (1994-1995), subsequently by Barney Singer, J.D. (1996-1998), and by Barbara Aranda-Naranjo, Ph.D., R.N. (1999-2000).

We also thank the valuable work of our Associate Editors on this volume. Trudy A. Larson, M.D., provided leadership for the Cooperative Agreement Steering Committee as its chair for all five years of the initiative and also served as the Principal Investigator for the project at the University of Nevada School of Medicine. Vivian B. Brown, Ph.D., served multiple roles in the Cooperative Agreement, including that of an Associate Director for the Evaluation and Dissemination Center and Principal Investigator of the PROTOTYPES WomensLink program for women living with HIV/AIDS. A. T. Panter, Ph.D., of the University of North Carolina Chapel Hill and a Senior Consultant to The Measurement Group was an integral member of the cross-cutting evaluation and dissemination team, providing extensive technical assistance to the grantees, particularly those focused on training healthcare providers to improve services for persons with HIV/AIDS. Drs. Larson, Brown, and Panter helped to ensure that the papers included in this special issue would be maximally useful and relevant for practitioners and researchers alike. In that respect, we also thank the contribution of the outside reviewers who reviewed these manuscripts and provided helpful comments and suggestions for the authors.

Finally, the production of this volume could not have been accomplished without the hard work of a number of staff at The Measurement Group. We thank Chermeen A. Elavia and Kimberly K. Ishihara for their assistance with manuscript preparation and word processing. We also wish to note the work of the late Diana E. Brief, Ph.D., who passed away unexpectedly before the completion of this project. Dr. Brief not only co-authored two papers in this volume, but also provided extensive technical assistance to all the projects throughout the course of the Cooperative Agreement to maximize the quality of data available to demonstrate the successes of these innovative service models.

REFERENCES

Huba, G. J., Melchior, L. A., Panter, A. T., and the HRSA/HAB SPNS Cooperative Agreement Steering Committee (2000a). Knowledge Item CA-Initiative Impact-07 from HRSA/HAB's SPNS Cooperative Agreements on Innovative Models of Care, The Measurement Group Knowledge Base on HIV/AIDS Care, Online at www.TheMeasurementGroup.com.

Huba, G. J., Melchior, L. A., Panter, A. T., & the HRSA/HAB SPNS Cooperative Agreement Steering Committee (2000b). The Measurement Group Knowledge Base on HIV/AIDS Care, Online at www.TheMeasurementGroup.com.

A National Program of AIDS Care Projects and Their Cross-Cutting Evaluation: The HRSA SPNS Cooperative Agreements

G. J. Huba, PhD
Lisa A. Melchior, PhD
A. T. Panter, PhD
Vivian B. Brown, PhD
Trudy A. Larson, MD

SUMMARY. As more people in the U.S. seek HIV care, the need has grown for demonstrated service models that address comprehensive needs. The Special Projects of National Significance (SPNS) Innovative Models of HIV Care Initiative funded by the Health Resources and

---

G. J. Huba and Lisa A. Melchior are affiliated with The Measurement Group, Culver City, CA. A. T. Panter is affiliated with the University of North Carolina at Chapel Hill and The Measurement Group. Vivian B. Brown is affiliated with PROTOTYPES, Culver City, CA. Trudy A. Larson is affiliated with the University of Nevada School of Medicine.

Address correspondence to: G. J. Huba, PhD, The Measurement Group, 5811A Uplander Way, Culver City, CA 90230 (E-mail: ghuba@TheMeasurementGroup. com).

Kimberly K. Ishihara and Chermeen A. Elavia provided manuscript production assistance.

This work was supported in part by the Health Resources and Services Administration (HRSA), HIV/AIDS Bureau (HAB), Special Projects of National Significance (SPNS) Grant No. 5 U90 HA 00030-05. This publication's contents are solely the responsibility of the authors and do not necessarily represent the official view of the funding agency.

The original modular evaluation strategy was designed by The Measurement Group and then enhanced by the Cooperative Agreement Projects and HRSA staff.

[Haworth co-indexing entry note]: "A National Program of AIDS Care Projects and Their Cross-Cutting Evaluation: The HRSA SPNS Cooperative Agreements." Huba, G. J. et al. Co-published simultaneously in *Drugs & Society* (The Haworth Press, Inc.) Vol. 16, No. 1/2, 2000, pp. 5-29; and: *Evaluating HIV/AIDS Treatment Programs: Innovative Methods and Findings* (ed: G. J. Huba et al.) The Haworth Press, Inc., 2000, pp. 5-29. Single or multiple copies of this article are available for a fee from The Haworth Document Delivery Service [1-800-342-9678, 9:00 a.m. - 5:00 p.m. (EST). E-mail address: getinfo@haworthpress inc.com].

Services Administration (HRSA) is an effort of 27 projects to jointly establish goals, develop common evaluation methods, and produce comparable and measurable outcomes. The projects have different service models, but share the goals of reducing barriers and improving access to quality HIV care. To evaluate the pooled effects of these models, a modular evaluation design (Huba & Melchior, 1995) was adopted. The use of shared evaluation protocols permits evaluation of the entire initiative, as well as the evaluation of project clusters with similar service delivery models. *[Article copies available for a fee from The Haworth Document Delivery Service: 1-800-342-9678. E-mail address: <getinfo@haworth pressinc.com> Website: <http://www.HaworthPress.com>]*

KEYWORDS. Program evaluation, HIV/AIDS, service demonstration projects, consensus process, community-based organizations, comprehensive healthcare models.

INTRODUCTION

On October 1, 1994, the Health Resources and Services Administration (HRSA) Special Projects of National Significance (SPNS) Program funded Innovative Models of HIV Care Initiative consisting of 27 Cooperative Agreement Projects, HRSA, and an Evaluation and Dissemination Center (EDC). The initiative included projects funded under four potential categories: those providing comprehensive medical care in a number of specific settings, those providing HIV services to "mobile" populations, those specifically designed to reduce barriers to care, and those providing training and educational models for improving the state of the art of HIV care in various treatment settings. An overview of these funding categories is included as Appendix I. The individual projects were funded for periods ranging from two to five years. A brief synopsis of each grantee funded through the cooperative agreement appears in Appendix II.

The funding mechanism for the HRSA SPNS Cooperative Agreement was selected for a variety of reasons. First, it was hoped that the cooperative agreement mechanism would help projects identify shared goals and objectives. Second, the cooperative agreement mechanism would enable projects to meet on a regular basis and share technical expertise among projects and with outside experts on programmatic concerns, staffing issues, and evaluation. Third, the cooperative agreement mechanism would enable a cross-cutting evaluation of major clusters of projects.

Structure and Decision-Making Processes of the Steering Committee for the Cooperative Agreement Projects

In its first year, the Steering Committee evolved a fairly straightforward decision making process which has worked well. Each of the 27 project representatives has one vote; the Evaluation and Dissemination Center representative has one vote; and the Health Resources and Services Administration representative has one vote. In addition to the chair of the Steering Committee, each of the Work Groups annually elects a chair. Together with the HRSA representative and the Director of the Evaluation and Dissemination Center, the chairs of the Work Groups form an ad hoc Executive Committee that holds telephone meetings–between scheduled, face-to-face Steering Committee meetings–usually to set the Steering Committee meeting agenda and rules. Day-to-day operations of the Steering Committee–including logistics, communications, and consultation–are guided by an Operations Committee consisting of the Steering Committee Chair, the HRSA representative, and the EDC Director. The EDC Director takes responsibility for ensuring that the decisions of the Operations Committee, the Executive Committee, and the larger Steering Committee are implemented. Figure 1 displays the group process and information sharing mechanism of the HRSA SPNS Cooperative Agreement Projects. The Steering Committee has found both of these mechanisms to be effective methods for managing its activities and for the sharing of project experiences.

FIGURE 1. Group Process and Information Sharing Mechanism of the SPNS Cooperative Agreement Projects

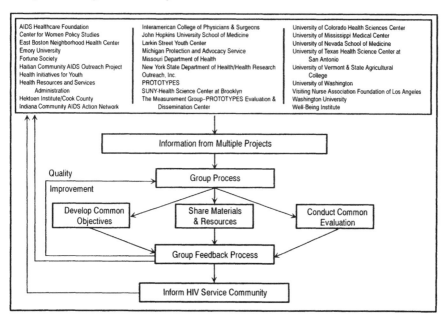

For the purposes of managing the cooperative agreements, sharing project expertise, and permitting cross-cutting evaluations, projects initially were assigned to one of five clusters based on similarities in methods, outcomes, and/or processes. The five working groups are summarized below.

- *Community-based organization models.* Six of the projects share, as a central theme, the goal of providing high-quality care for individuals with HIV who belong to groups that are traditionally underserved because of linguistic, cultural, racial, and economic barriers that prevent their full integration into the traditional hospital-based service system.
- *Comprehensive healthcare models.* Three projects are developing specialized medical care models within the context of a continuum of services in a medical clinic.
- *Capitated care models.* Five of the projects share, as a central theme, the study of the healthcare provided to individuals with HIV disease under models where the healthcare is capitated, or paid on a "flat fee" basis per patient per month. Each project shares the goals of determining costs for providing healthcare services to HIV/AIDS patients under a capitated care system and of ensuring that high quality care is provided under such a system, although the individual service models vary.
- *Infrastructure-advocacy models.* Seven projects in the Infrastructure-Advocacy group aim to increase the capacity of local health and social support service systems to provide appropriate, quality services for individuals with HIV. The projects in this group are using service system development methods through training and technical assistance to change the service provider infrastructure, as well as the community context in which services are delivered.
- *Training models.* While training is integral to almost all of the Cooperative Agreement Projects, seven have identified training among their most key elements.

This paper focuses on the overall evaluation strategy developed for the 27 HRSA SPNS Cooperative Agreement Projects, with a special emphasis on the projects of the Community-Based Organization Models and the Comprehensive Healthcare Work Group.

Common Evaluation Methods and Protocols

As a significant part of its activities during the first two years of funding, the Cooperative Agreement Steering Committee adopted a modular evaluation design that was suggested by the Evaluation and Dissemination Center (Huba & Melchior, 1995). In the modular evaluation design, standardized short forms of 1-2 pages were developed for a number of different functional evaluation questions. In collaboration between The Measurement Group and the Steering Committee, more than 70 modules were developed and implemented in the Cooperative Agreement Projects.

Table 1 summarizes each of the data collection modules utilized by the Cooperative Agreement Projects, provides reasons for their use, and gives the domains contained within each form. Additional information on these evaluation modules is given on the Internet at www.TheMeasurementGroup.com, where the actual forms have been posted.

Application of the modular approach. Many of the data collection modules summarized in Table 1 were developed in a scannable form that can either be faxed for automatic entry into the database, or mailed for manual scanning (Huba, Brown, & Melchior, 1995). Data collection forms, received either from the fax or from the scanner, are automatically appended to the project database at the EDC thus yielding data which is immediately up-to-date and readily available for analysis.

In addition to the short modules indicated above, longer modules were prepared as "standard" interview item sets, or as self-administered questionnaires. Data entry for these modules was by data entry shells developed in a standard database (Microsoft Access) and compiled so that the organization using the shell would not need to own a copy of the database software. The Evaluation and Dissemination Center provided these data entry shells to all project sites upon request to allow data entry at the site with transmission of the resulting data files to the Center. Alternately, data entry could be performed at the EDC.

For those projects that wished to collect information for a module using their standard database programs, the EDC arranged to receive a standard format data transfer approximately every 2-4 weeks. Sites were responsible for writing data to a standard format and sending it to the EDC on a regular schedule.

Modular evaluation design for the Community-Based Organization and Comprehensive Healthcare Work Groups. The majority of projects featured in this volume participated in either the Community-Based Organization or Comprehensive Healthcare Work Groups. Each of the Work Groups collaboratively developed and adopted common cross-cutting evaluation protocols to be able to pool their data and evaluate elements in common across their service models.

Especially among the Comprehensive Healthcare Projects–where a number of the projects have used databases which were previously constructed by their medical centers to capture patient characteristics and services–it has been agreed by these projects that the Evaluation and Dissemination Center would be permitted to judge whether there were sufficient indicators in the existing datasets that could be equated to these common requirements, or whether the existing data systems needed to be supplemented. Each of the

TABLE 1. Evaluation Modules Summary*

Module	Purpose	Content Domains
1. Demographics-Contact Form	• Code major demographic characteristics of clients. • Code risk-background factors. • Code reason for form. • Code referrals provided at contacts.	Race-ethnicity, gender, sexual orientation, age, reason for form, location, homeless status, HIV infection-retransmission risk factors, referrals to internal and external agencies and services.
2. Intervention Form	• Code units of client services. • Code providers. • Code purpose of client services. • Code referrals provided at interventions. • Code medications ordered or provided.	Types of service provided (outpatient medical, HIV testing/counseling, mental health, social supports, etc.), providers (physician, social worker, peer, etc.), purpose of services, referrals made to ancillary services, medications ordered or provided.
3. Presentations-Training Form	• Code type of presentation. • Code reason for presentation. • Code type of audience. • Code number of individuals of different demographic categories impacted.	Type of presentation (group prevention, agency recruitment, training, advocacy, policy), type of audience (educators, community members, service agencies, etc.), number of males and females of different age groups and ethnic-racial backgrounds in the audience.
4a. Individual Services Needed and Received Form 4b. Barriers and Facilitators Form	• Code services needed in the last six months and last month. • Code services received in the last six months and last month. • Code reason for not seeking-receiving needed services.	Types of services include drug detoxification, residential drug treatment, outpatient or day treatment substance abuse treatment, shelter, food or other basic needs, dentistry, outpatient/inpatient medical, HIV-related services, mental health, self-help, counseling, pharmacy, vocational training, case management, prenatal/pregnancy care, etc. Barriers include cost, accessibility, transportation, child care, staff disdain, language, coercion, disclosure concerns. Facilitators include caring staff, convenient location, and transportation.
5. Technical Assistance Summary Form	• Code major aspects of technical assistance. • Code reason for technical assistance. • Code type of audience for technical assistance. • Code number of individuals of different demographic categories impacted.	Type of technical assistance, type of audience, number of males and females of different age groups, ethnic-racial backgrounds, and professional service groups for whom assistance was given.
6. Technical Assistance Evaluation Form	• Code facets of satisfaction with the TA experience. • Rate value of TA for knowledge in a number of areas. • Rate pre-TA level of knowledge in a number of areas. • Rate post-TA levels of knowledge in a number of areas.	Overall satisfaction with the TA, specific dimensions of satisfaction (responsiveness, relevance, appropriateness, correct level, focus, efficiency), current knowledge levels, pre-TA knowledge levels, willingness to recommend TA for other projects and staff.

Module	Purpose	Content Domains
7. Agency Capacity Interview	• Code services currently provided. • Code services added in the last year. • Determine service capacities. • Assess likelihood of services expansion.	Capacity for a number of services including HIV inpatient and outpatient medical, mental health, substance abuse inpatient and outpatient treatment, shelter, basic needs, social services, family counseling, and ancillary services. Clients served. Likelihood of service expansion and barriers to expansion.
8. Agency Infrastructure-Attitudes Form	• Assess current attitudes about the area HIV service system. • Assess belief that system is integrated and enmeshed. • Code beliefs about equity and fairness in the service system. • Assess likelihood of referral to service sources. • Determine individual priorities for the use of HIV treatment and prevention funds.	Determines how the individual perceives the qualities of the overall HIV service system in the area, rate how resources should be allocated.
9. Agency Cohesiveness Rating Form	• Assess knowledge about other network services. • Assess willingness to make referrals to services. • Assess likelihood of receiving referrals from other services. • Assess overall connections to other services.	Determines how connected agencies in the same service system are to one another. Multidimensional scaling of perceived distances provides a mapping of the service system.
10. HIV Testing History Form	• Code times of previous testing. • Code previous testing history. • Code assistance rendered at previous testing times. • Code client belief or non-belief in previous HIV test results.	Develop a timeline of the HIV testing history, determine when first tested HIV-positive, services needed at time of testing, services received at time of testing, pre- and post-test counseling history.
11. Satisfaction with Services: General	• Code major aspects of satisfaction or dissatisfaction with services: general form for use with all populations.	Overall ratings of satisfaction with services, perception of service providers, importance rankings for service issues, perceived barriers, likelihood of future use and positive recommendations to family and peers.
12. Satisfaction with Services: Youth	• Code major aspects of satisfaction or dissatisfaction with services: special issues for youth form.	Covers specific issues for youth including service barriers and satisfaction with adult service providers, confidentiality from parents, appropriateness and relevance.
13. Satisfaction with Services: Older Adult	• Code major aspects of satisfaction or dissatisfaction with services: special issues for older adults form.	Covers specific issues for older adults including service barriers and satisfaction with providers, appropriateness and relevance.
14. Satisfaction with Services: Women	• Code major aspects of satisfaction or dissatisfaction with services: special issues for women form.	Covers specific issues for women including service barriers and satisfaction with providers, appropriateness and relevance, provisions for children and families, partner services.

TABLE 1 (continued)

Module	Purpose	Content Domains
15. Satisfaction with Services: Minorities	• Code major aspects of satisfaction or dissatisfaction with services: special issues for minorities form.	Covers specific issues for minorities including service barriers and satisfaction with providers, appropriateness and relevance, provisions for special language needs, cultural sensitivity to the client's background, multicultural viewpoint.
16. Standard Focus Group Characteristics Form	• Code participant characteristics in focus groups; client conclusions.	Covers client assessments of priorities for focus group topics. Standardized coding system for participant demographics.
17. Brief Health and Functioning Questionnaire– SF-21 Form	• Code participant health problems and syndromes diagnostic of, and related to, HIV disease. • Code general health levels and issues. • Code physical symptoms and problems. • Measure Health-Related Quality of Life.	Health items of major relevance to HIV disease. Includes CDC indicators of stage of HIV disease. May be used for repeatedly assessing progression of HIV disease.
18. Abbreviated HIV/AIDS Health Form–SF-21 Form only	• Code follow-up/repeated assessments of client health, progression of disease, and Health-Related Quality of Life.	Health items as above in an abbreviated format. Changes since last assessment.
19. HIV/AIDS Health Form: Women	• Code women-specific health issues. • Code issues such as child-rearing, birth control, pregnancy, etc., of particular relevance to a woman's health and functioning.	Items particularly related to women's health including reproductive history and medical syndromes and symptoms, STDs, other medical issues.
20. HIV/AIDS Risk Behaviors Form	• Code major issues of HIV risk and retransmission risk due to sexual contact. • Code major issues of HIV risk and retransmission risk due to injection drug use. • Code major issues of HIV risk and retransmission risk due to other means.	Number of sexual partners, sex acts with and without latex protection, injection drug use, hemophilia and other blood transfers, tendency to have sex while intoxicated or high, sex trade, sexual history of sex partners.
21. Weekly Program Census Form	• Method for capturing the weekly census on functional service units.	Weekly total census, demographic characteristics of census, method of collecting census.
22. Quality of Life Form	• Objective indicator of ability to engage in life activities such as being a partner, employment, attending recreational activities, etc. • Objective indicator of presence of sufficient resources to provide adequate standard of living. • Subjective indicator of self-perceived satisfaction with domain areas identified for objective indicators.	Rated ability to fully participate in and enjoy a large number of domains of activities including employment, being a partner, sexual relationships, recreation, travel, strenuous activity–exercise, enmeshment in the community. Checklist of activities participated in during the past month.

Module	Purpose	Content Domains
23. Follow-up Quality of Life Form	• Follow-up version of Quality of Life Form designed for repeated use. • Changes in Quality of Life since previous assessment.	Abbreviated versions of Quality of Life items listed above. Changes in QOL are specifically coded.
24. Substance Abuse History Form	• Standardized measure of lifetime and current substance abuse including both injection and non-injection routes of administration.	Ever used, use in last 6 months, use in last month of: alcohol, marijuana, cocaine, heroin, crack, speedballs, amphetamines, PCP, LSD, other hallucinogens, barbiturates, other drugs. Injection drug use. Needle sharing/cleaning behaviors.
25. Activities of Daily Living Form	• Standardized measure to assess current ability to conduct standard living activities including meal preparation, use of telephone, handling finances, taking medication, etc.	Checklist of clients' ability to do daily life activities: dressing, preparing meals, driving an automobile, attending work, etc. Designed for repeated assessments, possibly daily.
26. Current Psychological Distress Form	• Standardized measure of psychological distress comparable to major studies conducted over 15 years throughout the U.S.: Center for Epidemiological Studies Depression Scale (CES-D).	In last seven days: depressed, moody, blue, lonely, etc.
27. Residential Services Daily Services Form	• Codes daily activities and services received in residential facility including treatment programs and hospices.	Number of minutes spent in groups, therapy, counseling, psychotherapy, vocational training; visits to physician, psychiatrist, other professionals.
28. Outpatient Services Daily Services Form	• Code daily activities and services received in outpatient facility and services.	Number of minutes spent in groups, therapy, individual counseling, psychotherapy, vocational training; visits to physician, psychiatrist, other professionals.
29. Standardized Focus Group Instructions	• Standardized specifications for conducting focus groups. • Suggested format for reporting focus group results. • Suggested qualitative and quantitative questions for focus groups.	Standard grid for eliciting focus group free-responses, demographic items to code focus group participants, facilitator form to code reason for focus group and major dynamics, standardized methods for ranking alternatives.
30. Standardized Instructions for Case Studies	• Standardized specifications for selecting clients for case studies. • Suggested format for reporting case study results. • Suggested domains to be discussed in case studies. • Suggested quantitative indices to be included in case studies.	Standard outline for case studies including patient background, major medical problems, health history, prior maximum levels of social and psychological adjustment, current psychological impairment, current physical impairment, quality of life, and ancillary problems (substance abuse, violence, homelessness, etc.). Includes information about progression of disease, quality of life, and service utilization history.
31. Sexual Behaviors Form	• Code current sexual practices including partners.	Number of current partners of both sexes, total sexual partners in past years, sexual partners of both sexes who were injection drug users, sex with male and female partners with and without latex protection, types of sexual practices.

TABLE 1 (continued)

Module	Purpose	Content Domains
32. Abuse History	• Code history of physical abuse. • Code levels of physical abuse. • Code history of sexual abuse. • Code current levels of sexual abuse. • Code admitted behaviors as abuser.	Lifetime and current indicators of physical and sexual abuse from parents, other family, and strangers. Admitted abuse against others.
33. Self-Esteem	• Code current levels of self-esteem.	Use major, multidimensional self-esteem scale. (Rosenberg)
34. Partner Disclosure Risk Form	• Code likelihood of being recipient of partner violence if HIV status is disclosed.	Indicators of potential partner psychological, verbal, and physical violence at disclosure of HIV status.
35. Homelessness Index	• Code stability of current housing situations. • Code history of housing stability.	Time history of places lived and with whom, log of places slept in the last year and month, use of shelters, ability to support a permanent home.
36. Family Composition Form	• Code current and past family members. • Code major aspects of family functioning including cohesiveness, support, stability.	History of children, partners, siblings, parents, extended family. Ratings of current family problems and strengths.
37. Personality Test Battery	• Code major dimensions of psychological functioning.	Basic Personality Inventory. Includes dimensions for thought disorder, depression, alienation, denial, and social introversion.
38. Suicide Probability	• Standardized indicator of suicide potential.	Suicide Probability Scale.
39. Emotional Functioning Battery	• Standardized measure of present mood and emotional state.	Profile of Mood States or alternative.
40. Cognitive-Neurological Test Battery	• Screening test for neuropsychological impairment.	Screening test for the Luria-Nebraska Neuropsychological Battery (LNNB-ST). Indicates likely pathology in a full neuropsychological work-up.
41. Standardized Nutrition Schedule	• Standardized nutrition recording form permitting an estimate of calories consumed.	Overall schedule of food consumed, total calorie estimate, hunger, desire to eat.
42. Psychosocial Observations Form	• Code perceived level of cognitive, social, intellectual functioning. • Code appearance, obvious behavior problems, emotional state. • Code manner of speaking.	Ratings of functioning levels; behavioral descriptions of emotional state, appearance, stated problems, inferred problems, manner of speaking, possible intoxication, disorganization.
43. Clinical Observations Form	• Code levels of behavioral, mental, and health problems. • Code unusual incidents. • Code changes in status.	Ratings of clinical problem levels conducted by clinical staff. Goes beyond psychosocial observations by requiring trained clinical inference.
44. Progress Ratings Form	• Code progress of deterioration, HIV disease, or adherence to treatment regimens. • Code barriers to progress. • Code client satisfaction with progress.	Ratings of overall progress including changes.

Module	Purpose	Content Domains
45. Life Stressors Form	• Standard measure of the presence of significant sources of life stress.	Checklist of major life stressors and valence associated with each.
46. Social Supports Form	• Standard measure of the presence and importance of sources for social support.	Ratings of support from partner, children, parents, other family, HIV-positive individuals, church, employer, male friends, female friends, etc.
47. Coping	• Standard indicators of modes of coping with stress and illness.	Assessment of coping through denial, projection, discounting, emotional leveling, and other methods. Coping will be assessed both as a general theme and in terms of coping with HIV disease.
48. Resources to Deal with HIV Disease	• Assessment of financial resources to cope with HIV disease. • Health insurance, disability benefits, "negative" life insurance benefits.	Income from work, relatives, annuities, disability insurance, selling death benefits. Self perceived adequacy of these sources of income to provide adequate quality of life and medical care.
49. Staff Characteristics Form	• Major demographic characteristics of staff service provider. • Experiential background of service provider. • Educational background of service provider. • Major "treatment philosophy" of service provider.	Staff race-ethnicity, age, gender, sexual orientation, similarity to target groups (HIV-positive, drug abuser, mental health diagnosis), educational background, ratings of agreement with treatment practices and philosophy items.
50. Future Plans Form	• Perceived desire and likelihood engaging in major life events in the next 12 months.	Ratings of perceived likelihood and desirability of life events including holding a job, parenting, having a child, travel, forming new friendships, doing volunteer activities, etc.
51. Referral Form	• Codes referrals made to participating social service agencies.	Tracking of referrals for social services, mental health, substance abuse treatment, basic needs services.
52. Cost Effectiveness Guidelines	• Guidelines for calculating cost effectiveness statistics.	Standardized directions and definitions for calculating cost-effectiveness.
53. Trainee Characteristics Form	• Code major demographic characteristics of trainees. • Code professional background. • Code prior experience/knowledge of HIV/AIDS issues.	Ethnic-racial, age, types of professional training and degrees, professional identification and licensure, experience with clinical aspects of HIV/AIDS, experience with HIV/AIDS prevention techniques.
54. Trainee Reactions to Training Form	• Code major facets of satisfaction with the training experience. • Code satisfaction with trainers. • Rate value of training for knowledge in a number of HIV/AIDS-related areas.	Satisfaction with training, connection with trainers, perceived utility of information-skills presented, value of training and relevance for own job.
55. Trainee Reactions to Training Follow-up Form	• Short version of above used for temporal follow-up.	Satisfaction with training, connection with trainers, perceived utility of information-skills presented, value of training and relevance for own job.

TABLE 1 (continued)

Module	Purpose	Content Domains
56. Trainer Characteristics Form	• Major demographic characteristics of trainer. • Experiential background of trainer. • Educational background of trainer. • Major "philosophy" of trainer.	Trainer race-ethnicity, age, gender, sexual orientation, similarity to target groups (HIV-positive, drug abuser, mental health diagnosis), educational background, ratings of agreement with practices and philosophy items.
57. Training Evaluation Form: Knowledge, Attitudes, Comfort	• Code major areas of HIV/AIDS knowledge. • Code attitudes toward HIV/AIDS and related conditions. • Code self-perceived comfort dealing with topics related to HIV/AIDS.	Standardized scale of HIV/AIDS knowledge for healthcare professionals. Standardized scale of attitudes toward HIV/AIDS and related conditions. Standardized scale of degree of comfort in addressing HIV/AIDS topics.
58. Training Evaluation Form: Knowledge, Attitudes, Comfort Follow-up	• Short version of above used for temporal follow-up.	Alternate and/or abbreviated form of Module 57.
59. Training Evaluation Form: Standardized Scenarios for HIV/AIDS Training	• Standardized scenarios in AIDS Care, HIV Prevention, Referrals, Related Conditions-Diseases, Current Therapies, Needs of Special Groups. • Code knowledge, attitudes, skills, comfort.	Brief (1-2 paragraph) constructed to assess major issues in patient care, HIV prevention, and related issues. Each scenario followed by 6-12 questions assessing knowledge, attitudes, skills, and comfort in dealing with the topic.
60. Training Evaluation Form: Standardized Scenarios for HIV/AIDS Training Alternate	• Alternate versions of above used for temporal follow-up.	Brief (1-2 paragraph) constructed to assess major issues in patient care, HIV prevention, and related issues. Each scenario followed by 6-12 questions assessing knowledge, attitudes, skills, and comfort in dealing with the topic.
61. Hotline Client Background and Referral Form	• Codes client calls to a hotline or agency when such calls constitute a service. • Codes referrals made to participating social service agencies.	Tracking of client characteristics and nature of the call. Tracking of referrals for social services, mental health, substance abuse treatment, basic needs services, etc.
62. Chart Review Standards	• Codes major variables related to physician and other healthcare provider practices from medical chart. • Codes major variables related to client stage of HIV disease from medical chart.	Codes HIV-related conditions and other health problems; major clinical markers such as CD4 count and viral load.
63. HIV Status Report, AIDS Related Variables	• Codes major HIV disease related variables on a single form. • Items taken from HRSA Uniform Reporting System (URS).	CDC-defined disease stage, CD4 count, source of status, exposure category, TB status.
64. Self Efficacy Scale	• Codes feelings of mastery.	Standardized scale with known reliability and validity.

	Module	Purpose	Content Domains
65.	Acceptance of Disease Scale	• Codes acceptance of HIV disease. • Codes ability to view the successes and positive impact of one's life. • Codes feelings that previously unresolved issues related to family and friends have been resolved.	Ways of demonstrating acceptance of diagnosis and health status.
66.	Training Evaluation Form: Characterization of Training Form	• Codes training topics. • Codes training methods. • Codes units of training.	Type of presentation, type of training methods. [Module 3 is preferred.]
67.	General Well Being Scale	• Codes feelings of well being in a number of different areas of life.	Standardized scale by Andrews and Withey and used in General Social Survey since 1976. National data available. Used in hundreds of studies.
68.	Program Discharge Form	• Codes discharge date. • Codes reasons for program discharge.	Reasons for discharge including voluntary and involuntary withdrawal from the program, movement from service area, death.
69.	Suggested standards for ethnographic research	• Defines major issues and standards for ethnographic research.	Differentiates ethnographic research from other forms of qualitative research.
70.	Short Health Rating Form	• The purpose of this module is to make a quick assessment of health at a given point in time.	Codes client's rating of overall health, CD4 count, and Karnofsky rating.
71.	Medical Health Form	• The purpose of this module is to assess medical health conditions that are related to HIV disease.	Codes HIV-related conditions such as PCP, MAI, TB, and other health problems.
72.	Missed Visit/ Appointment Form	• The purpose of this module is to record missed appointments or office visits by a client. This is a key issue in tracking adherence to program advice.	Codes type of appointment missed and reason missed.
73.	Karnofsky and Disease Stage Scale	• The purpose of this form is to code stage of disease, CD4 count, and Karnofsky ratings for a client.	Graphically represents stage of disease as a function of CD4 count; includes annotated Karnofsky rating scale.
74.	Urinalysis Report Form	• The purpose of this form is to record the results of urinalysis that may be conducted as part of monitoring for use of alcohol or other drugs.	Codes substances detected and confirmed via urinalysis. Does not specify which assay method is used in the urinalysis.
75.	Disclosure Questionnaire	• The purpose of this module is to record which close friend and service providers the individual has informed about his/her HIV.	Codes individuals who are close to the person, individuals who were told about client HIV, reasons for not disclosing, and whether or not service providers have been told.
76.	Service Use by Family Interview	• The purpose of this module is to record persons living in the household and the services they needed and/or received.	Code information about members of the household and service use by current and past family members.

TABLE 1 (continued)

Module	Purpose	Content Domains
77. Training Evaluation Form for National AIDS Update	• The purpose of this form is to evaluate the youth component of the National AIDS Update Conference workshops.	Codes educational background, types of professional training and degrees, comfort and knowledge with workshop topics, satisfaction with workshop, usefulness of information presented, quality of workshop and relevance for own job.
78. Key Informant Interviews, Comprehensive Healthcare Projects	• The purpose of this interview is to elicit feedback from stakeholders in each of three comprehensive healthcare service delivery programs for persons living with HIV/AIDS.	Codes information about the progress of these projects in areas such as patient recruitment and retention, accessibility, quality of care, education and training, consumer involvement, development of service networks, and information dissemination.
79. Adolescent Protease Inhibitor Therapy	• The purpose of this interview is to gauge a patient's overall adherence to protease inhibitor therapy.	Codes information about the number of medications a patient is taking, provider-patient interactions, protease inhibitor history, participation in clinical trials, medication side effects experienced, attitudes about medication, social interactions.
80. Collaborative Agencies Evaluation Form	• The purpose of this form is to assess how well collaborating agencies work with one another.	Codes information about agency involvement, professional background, usefulness of agency's trainings, collaboration/referral network improvements, changes/improvement in services provided, overall satisfaction with agency.
81. Nutrition Clinic Evaluation Form	• The purpose of this interview is to gather information about the experiences and services received by clients at an HIV nutrition clinic.	Codes information about client background, health ratings, ratings of perceived importance of various nutrition services, barriers to receiving nutrition services, involvement in nutrition visits.
82. Training Impact Follow-Up Interview	• The purpose of this interview is to obtain information about the effectiveness of trainings on systems change and changes in patient care.	Codes information about trainees': major demographic characteristics, professional background, satisfaction with training, perceived effect of trainings on changes in patient care and systems change.

* Adapted from the SPNS Cooperative Agreement Evaluation Module Summary Book (Huba & Melchior, 1995).

projects agreed that if it was not using the agreed upon modules that it would make its databases available to the EDC to equate, and if needed, to supplement its datasets. That is, it was not required that the exact paper modules in the Cooperative Agreement Module Book be implemented using standard forms, but the projects were required to collect the indicators in a way to be functionally equivalent to those forms, and to make the data available to the EDC. The EDC was charged with combining the datasets into comparable indicators. The EDC was also given the latitude by the Work Group to make judgments about the equivalency of local data collection methods from site-to-site.

Table 2 summarizes the evaluation design for the Community-Based Organization Work Group. Because this Work Group primarily provides psychosocial services, the cross-cutting evaluation data elements reflect that focus. The members of this Work Group agreed to collect the information on Modules 1 (Demographics-Contact), 2B (Psychosocial Intervention Services), 4A (Services Needed and Received), 4B (Barriers and Facilitators), 11 (Client Satisfaction), 17 (Brief Health and Functioning; first page, or equivalently Module 18), 51 (Referral), and 68 (Discharge/Departure). The specifications in the table were for the absolute minimum frequency with which the indicators should be collected. It was recommended that the data be collected much more often if possible.

TABLE 2. Community-Based Organization Work Group Evaluation Design

Module Number	Module Name	Purpose	Minimum Frequency of Administration
1	Demographic-Contact Form	To record characteristics of patients who are admitted to services.	At intake and updated in first 90 days.
2B	Psychosocial Intervention Services Form	To record psychosocial services provided to clients.	Every intervention or when services are administered (can be completed per visit or on a daily basis).
4A	Services Needed and Received	To collect needs expressed and services received by the client.	At intake and every 6 months.
4B	Barriers and Facilitators Form	To collect client perceptions of barriers and facilitators to services.	At intake and every 6 months.
11	Client Satisfaction Survey	To assess client satisfaction with services.	Every 6 months.
17	Brief Health and Functioning Questionnaire	To assess health related quality of life during the course of HIV disease.	At intake and every 6 months.
51	Referral Form	To have a standardized way of tracking service referrals that are made to collateral and cooperating agencies.	As they occur.
68	Discharge/Program Departure Form	To code a client's discharge from the SPNS-funded program along with the reason(s) for the discharge.	As needed.

Table 3 shows the evaluation design for the Comprehensive Healthcare Work Group. As can be seen, a number of process and outcome data elements were the same as those collected by the Community-Based Organization Work Group, such as Client Characteristics (Module 1), Psychosocial Services (Module 2B), Psychological Distress (Module 26), Client Satisfaction (Module 11), and Health-Related Quality of Life (Modules 17/18). However, the Comprehensive Healthcare projects also collected medical indicator data such as Medical Service Encounters (Module 2A), Medications Provided (Module 2C), and Medical Health Indicators (Module 71). The Community-Based Organization projects were also encouraged to collect medical indicator data when available, although such data were not required elements in their pooled evaluation design.

The following provides additional information about evaluation modules collected by projects in both the Community-Based Organization (CBO) and Comprehensive Healthcare (Comp Care) Work Groups.

- Module 1 (Demographics-Contact) was designed as a program enrollment form. Since not all data may be available immediately upon enrollment of the patient, data may be completed and updated during the first 90 days of services. (CBO, Comp Care)
- Module 2A (Medical Intervention Services Form) was designed to capture the services provided within the medical components of the service at each encounter. The Work Group agreed that either a "per encounter" format may be used, or data may be coded so as to summarize a single day of services. The EDC was charged with making data across sites comparable. (Comp Care)
- Module 2B (Psychosocial Intervention Services Form) was designed to capture the services provided within the psychosocial components of the service at each encounter. The Work Group agreed that either a "per encounter" format may be used, or data may be coded so as to summarize a single day of services. The EDC was charged with making data across sites comparable. (CBO, Comp Care)
- Module 2C (Medications Ordered or Provided) was intended to be unique to all sites. Because the sites could not agree on a comparable format, it was decided that pharmaceutical records from each project would be submitted to the EDC in electronic form as they are obtained either from medical clinic records or from a third party pharmaceutical provider. The EDC was charged with summarizing these forms into a comparable format for all projects. (Comp Care)
- Module 4A (Services Needed and Received Form) was designed to document the needs expressed and services received by the clients. The EDC recommended that this information be collected as often as possible since needs may change over time. (CBO)

- Module 4B (Barriers and Facilitators Form) was designed to document clients' perceptions of barriers and facilitators to receiving services. The EDC recommended that this information be collected as often as possible since barriers may change over time. (CBO)
- Module 11 (Client Satisfaction) was to be administered a minimum of one time per year to all patients. The EDC recommended that this be completed quarterly or at a minimum of every six months. (CBO, Comp Care)
- Module 17 (Brief Health and Functioning) was designed to be administered every six months. Projects could opt to use Module 18, which is the first half of the instrument, since the information on the last half was captured in other ways. (CBO, Comp Care)
- Module 51 (Referral Form) was designed to be administered whenever a referral was made to services. This module provided a mechanism by which service referrals could be tracked. (CBO)
- Module 68 (Discharge-Departure) was used to code the reasons that a patient was no longer receiving services. (CBO, Comp Care)
- Module 71 (Medical Health Form) was designed to be administered as appropriate, but at least every six months. The EDC was charged with combining the information from projects collected in different time durations into a comparable time frame. The EDC recommended that this information be collected as often as possible. (Comp Care)

CONCLUSION

As the number of people seeking HIV care in the U.S. has grown, the demand has increased not only for medical care, but also for a wide range of supportive services. This in turn has increased the need for demonstrated and tested HIV/AIDS service delivery models that can address a comprehensive set of needs. By grouping projects by a common programmatic element for evaluation using common modules, as much comparable data as possible may be obtained from each of these projects. Furthermore, through the development and administration of these very brief modules, data collection efforts for the projects are customized by including those modules that fit the specific goals and objectives of the project. In addition, the use of common data collection forms permits the cross-cutting evaluation necessary for the HRSA SPNS Innovative Model of HIV Care Initiative as a whole.

As evaluation results emerge from the Cooperative Agreement Projects, outlets such as this volume are an excellent opportunity to disseminate the findings from these innovative models of HIV care. The web site of The Measurement Group at www.TheMeasurementGroup.com is also a key element in disseminating information about evaluation designs, methods, and results from these service delivery models. The web site includes summaries

TABLE 3. Comprehensive Healthcare Work Group Evaluation Design

Module Number	Module Name	Purpose	Minimum Frequency of Administration
1	Demographic-Contact Form	To record characteristics of patients who are admitted to services.	At intake and updated in first 90 days.
2A	Medical Intervention Services Form	To record medical services provided to patients.	Every medical intervention or when medical services are administered (can be completed per visit or on a daily basis).
2B	Psychosocial Intervention Services Form	To record psychosocial services provided to patients.	Every psychosocial intervention or when psychosocial services are administered (can be completed per visit or on a daily basis).
2C	Medications Ordered or Provided	To document medication ordered for or provided to patients.	Whenever medications are ordered for or dispensed to patient.
11	Client Satisfaction Survey	To assess patient satisfaction with services.	Once a year.
17	Brief Health and Functioning Questionnaire	To assess health related quality of life during the course of HIV disease.	At intake and every 6 months (if patient's CD4-cell count is below 75, it is recommended–but not required–that data be collected every 3 months).
68	Discharge/Program Departure Form	To code a patient's discharge from the SPNS-funded program along with the reason(s) for the discharge.	As needed.
71	Medical Health Form	To document medically related health conditions during the course of HIV disease.	At intake and every 6 months (if patient's CD4-cell count is below 75, it is recommended–but not required–that data be collected every 3 months).

of the evaluation designs for each of the Cooperative Agreement Work Groups, electronic versions of the data collection modules, and many related resources. Also housed in the web site of The Measurement Group is a Knowledge Base on Innovative HIV/AIDS Care models. The Knowledge Base includes cross-cutting results from the Cooperative Agreement Projects, and is updated continuously as new results become available. By placing these resources on the Internet, it is anticipated that others wishing to evaluate similar programs may export the evaluation methods used in this multisite evaluation to other settings.

REFERENCES

Huba, G. J. & Melchior, L. A. (1995). Evaluation module summary for the SPNS Cooperative Agreement Steering Committee.

Huba, G. J., Brown, V. B., & Melchior, L. A. (1995). Fax-in forms as a technology for evaluating community projects: An evaluation of HIV risk reduction. *Educational and Psychological Measurement, 55* (1), 75-83.

APPENDIX I

Overview of Categories for the SPNS Innovative Models of HIV Care Initiative

The following table shows the major categories under which projects were funded.

1. Provide a comprehensive primary care service delivery or specialized medical care system within one distinct environment or setting relating to one of the following subcategories:

    (1a) To develop and evaluate the effectiveness of primary care as part of a managed care plan or a comprehensive, coordinated care system;
    (1b) To test the feasibility of providing comprehensive HIV services as part of a capitated reimbursement system;
    (1c) To add primary care services to an intermediate level of care;
    (1d) To develop a comprehensive continuum of care in a defined rural area;
    (1e) To develop a service delivery model for effectively managing the medical and substance abuse treatment needs of adolescents with Stage III or IV HIV infection; or
    (1f) To develop a service delivery model for women with HIV emphasizing coordination of related services.

2. Provide a coordinated delivery of HIV health and support services to specific "mobile" populations in the United States. (No projects were approved in this category for funding.)

3. Reduction of cultural, linguistic, and/or organizational barriers to care in a geographically defined area as it relates to one of the following subcategories:

    (3a) For an underserved population by addressing their access to care issues through organizational collaboration and inclusion in policy development;
    (3b) For an ethnic group that faces both linguistic and cultural barriers;
    (3c) For active substance abusers; or
    (3d) For individuals or special populations experiencing HIV-based discrimination.

4. Provider training and education models for increasing, improving, or updating knowledge about HIV infection and its treatment in rural, correctional, or mental health settings.

APPENDIX II

SPNS Cooperative Agreement Projects

AIDS Healthcare Foundation (Los Angeles, California)

Grant title. *Test the Feasibility of Providing Comprehensive HIV Services Under a Capitated Reimbursement System.*
Description. AHF is demonstrating that an enhanced, capitated, managed healthcare approach to providing HIV/AIDS care will produce fewer opportunistic infections, fewer and shorter hospitalizations, better compliance with medical treatment, and an overall longer life span, including a better quality of life for HIV/AIDS diagnosed populations.

Center for Community Health, Education, and Research/Haitian Community AIDS Outreach Project (Dorchester, Massachusetts)

Grant title. *Enhanced Innovative Community and Hospital-Based Case Management Program.*
Description. The Center for Community Health, Education and Research/ Haitian AIDS Project (CCHER/HAP) of Dorchester, Massachusetts is seeking to enhance its current community and hospital-based HIV/AIDS case management system, to offer one-on-one intensive counseling sessions and educational training, and to develop a culturally competent risk reduction curriculum for its target population of Haitians.

Center for Women Policy Studies (Washington, District of Columbia)

Grant title. *Metro DC Collaborative for Women with HIV.*
Description. In collaboration with PROTOTYPES, the Center for Women Policy Studies' project–the Metro DC Collaborative for Women with HIV–is reducing organizational barriers to care for women with HIV through organizational collaboration and inclusion of women with HIV, their providers, and advocates in policy development.

East Boston Neighborhood Health Center (East Boston, Massachusetts)

Grant title. *Development of an HIV/AIDS Service Delivery Model.*
Description. By exploring the feasibility of developing three separate, capitated reimbursement rates for patients who will be appropriately grouped

according to clinical diagnosis–HIV-positive asymptomatic, HIV-positive symptomatic, and CDC AIDS–this project is developing a cost-efficient, community-based HIV/AIDS care plan.

Emory University (Atlanta, Georgia)

Grant title. *HIV Training for Georgia Correctional Providers.*

Description. The grantee is developing, testing, and evaluating educational models for increasing, improving, and updating knowledge about HIV infection and treatment for Georgia's correctional healthcare providers.

Fortune Society (New York, New York)

Grant title. *Discharge Planning and Case Management for Latino and Latina Prisoners Who Are HIV-Positive and Symptomatic.*

Description. The Fortune Society delivers culturally and linguistically appropriate services to Hispanic women and men prisoners and releasees who are HIV-positive and symptomatic in New York City jails and New York state prisons.

Health Initiatives for Youth (San Francisco, California)

Grant title. *Youth AIDS/HIV Community Training Project (YouthACT).*

Description. This project helps health and human service providers offer developmentally and culturally appropriate care for HIV-affected youth and young adults ages 12-25 living in the San Francisco Bay area.

Hektoen Institute for Medical Research/Cook County HIV Primary Care Center (Chicago, Illinois)

Grant title. *Illinois Maternal and Child Health Integrated Project.*

Description. The project is working to insure HIV education, counseling and testing by consent in all family planning and perinatal sites in Cook County to guarantee on-going care for identified women living with HIV and their families.

Indiana Community AIDS Action Network (Indianapolis, Indiana)

Grant Title. *Indiana HIV Advocacy Program.*

Description. The project targets African Americans and men who have sex with men to increase their utilization of advocacy services and, therefore, reduce barriers to healthcare access and discriminatory practices encountered in healthcare settings, employment, housing, public accommodations, governmental services, criminal justice, social/domestic relations, and insurance.

Interamerican College of Physicians and Surgeons (New York, New York)

Grant title. *Expanding Access to Healthcare Services for Hispanic HIV-Infected/STD Patients by Promoting Early Intervention, Screening, and Counseling Among Hispanic Physicians.*

Description. ICPS expands access to healthcare services for HIV-positive Hispanic populations by increasing, through training, the number of Hispanic healthcare providers active in screening, testing, counseling and managing their patients at-risk or already HIV infected.

Johns Hopkins University School of Medicine (Baltimore, Maryland)

Grant title. *Johns Hopkins–Medicaid AIDS Capitated Care Program.*
Description. The project is reducing the financial barriers to adequate care for AIDS patients and to improve the comprehensiveness of their care while containing costs to the insurer and reducing uncompensated costs to the provider.

Larkin Street Services (San Francisco, California)

Grant title. *HIV Service Delivery Model for Homeless Youth and Young Adults, 16 to 26 Years of Age, with CDC Defined Stage III and IV AIDS.*
Description. This project provides emergency housing, comprehensive primary medical care and psychosocial support services for homeless youth living with HIV/AIDS and will establish an "Assisted Care Facility" that will consist of a twelve-unit assisted living and long-term care facility.

Michigan Protection and Advocacy Service (Lansing, Michigan)

Grant title. *HIV/AIDS Advocacy Program–Community Advocate Training Program.*
Description. Michigan Protection and Advocacy has expanded its HIV/ AIDS Advocacy Program by providing consumers with legal representation and by providing training to attorneys, consumers, and service providers in African American, gay and lesbian, and rural communities regarding HIV legal issues.

Missouri Department of Health (Jefferson City, Missouri)

Grant title. *Integrated Care for Individuals with HIV/AIDS, Mental Illness, and/or Substance Abuse Problems.*
Description. This project develops and implements an "Integrated Model of Care" for individuals with HIV/AIDS that are diagnosed with a mental illness and/or substance abuse problems.

New York State Department of Health/Health Research (Albany, New York)

Grant title. *New York State Managed Care Demonstration Project for HIV-Infected Persons.*
Description. This project involves a dynamic data collection effort to generate information related to cost, utilization and access to care as persons with HIV/AIDS transition from fee-for-service to a managed care environment.

Outreach, Inc. (Atlanta, Georgia)

Grant title. *Safe Place.*

Description. Outreach's project, Safe Place, uses a peer counselor and street team model to expand enrollment and enhance retention of substance abusers with HIV in primary care by opening a satellite facility within an African American neighborhood near downtown Atlanta.

PROTOTYPES (Culver City, California)

Grant title. *PROTOTYPES WomensLink: Reduction of Barriers to HIV/ AIDS Care.*

Description. This project consists of a store-front meeting place where active substance abusing women with HIV/AIDS and their families are able to access a comprehensive, "seamless" continuum of services.

SUNY Health Science Center at Brooklyn (Brooklyn, New York)

Grant title. *The Brooklyn Service Model.*

Description. This project is reducing the frequency of perinatal transmission of HIV, enhancing access to care for women with HIV, and disseminating successful models of early identification and care.

University of Colorado Health Sciences Center (Denver, Colorado)

Grant title. *Educating Rural Providers to Improve HIV Services.*

Description. The project is evaluating the impact and cost effectiveness of three educational methodologies designed to increase service delivery to at-risk and HIV-seropositive individuals in rural areas.

University of Mississippi Medical Center (Jackson, Mississippi)

Grant title. *HIV Early Intervention for Mississippi Community Health Centers.*

Description. The project enhances the capacity of healthcare providers in rural clinics to diagnose and treat asymptomatic HIV disease by providing clinical training for those providers with a computer-based distance learning system.

University of Nevada School of Medicine (Reno, Nevada)

Grant title. *Early Nutrition Intervention in HIV and AIDS.*

Description. The project is based on the association between weight loss and nutritional deficiency in HIV-infected persons and, therefore, provides comprehensive nutrition assessment and intervention services to relatively healthy HIV-infected individuals.

University of Texas Health Science Center at San Antonio (San Antonio, Texas)

Grant title. *SPNS Family Unit Project for South Texas (Project SALUD).*

Description. The project provides a mechanism for urban and rural communities to build upon existing strengths and capacities for continued development of a comprehensive, family-centered continuum of care for HIV/AIDS women, children and their families living in South Texas.

University of Vermont & State Agricultural College (Burlington, Vermont)

Grant title. *Healthcare Delivery for People with HIV/AIDS in Rural Vermont.*

Description. The project has developed three state-of-the-art rural community HIV satellite clinics in Vermont that supplement services currently being provided by the state's only other comprehensive HIV clinic.

University of Washington (Seattle, Washington)

Grant title. *Psychiatric Management of HIV/AIDS Patients with Delirium.*

Description. The project trains and educates primary care providers, mental health staff, and volunteers to develop, test, and evaluate strategies for increasing, improving, and updating knowledge about HIV neuropsychiatric illness with specific emphasis on delirium and its treatment.

Visiting Nurse Association Foundation (Los Angeles, California)

Grant title. *AIDS Special Care Program: A Capitation Baseline Demonstration Project.*

Description. The project compares service utilization, costs of care, quality of life, and patient outcomes of approximately 1,000 AIDS-infected clients under a fee-for-service Medicare/Medicaid reimbursement system and a condition-based Medicare/Medicaid capitated hospice.

Washington University (St. Louis, Missouri)

Grant title. *Special Care Center for Women with HIV.*

Description. The project has developed a special care unit for women with HIV in a 12 county area around St. Louis that identifies women with HIV at an earlier stage, increases their access to services and clinical trials, provides support services, decreases preventable opportunistic infections and vertical HIV transmission, and improves quality of life.

Well-Being Institute (Detroit, Michigan)

Grant title. *Well-Being Institute Women's Intervention Program.*

Description. The program is a comprehensive, nursing-based intervention program designed for women HIV-positive substance abusers to decrease barriers to care, assist women to become drug free, provide housing for the women and their children, and work with them on a revenue-generating, entrepreneurial activity, making and selling crafts.

The Measurement Group-PROTOTYPES (Culver City, California)

Grant title. *Evaluation and Dissemination Center: SPNS HIV Service Delivery Grants.*

Description. The Measurement Group-PROTOTYPES consortium provides consultation and technical support services to grantees, which include components of centralized data entry/management, statistical and management information reports, and information dissemination functions.

Conceptual Issues in Implementing and Using Evaluation in the "Real World" Setting of a Community-Based Organization for HIV/AIDS Services

G. J. Huba, PhD
Vivian B. Brown, PhD
Lisa A. Melchior, PhD
Chi Hughes, MSW
A. T. Panter, PhD

SUMMARY. This paper examines a number of conceptual issues inherent in conducting program evaluation and research within a community-based organization (CBO). The paper considers three major types of issues that must be addressed in the evaluation of community-based organizations: (1) programmatic considerations CBOs face; (2) major evaluation design considerations; and (3) how the program and evalua-

---

G. J. Huba and Lisa A. Melchior are affiliated with The Measurement Group, Culver City, CA. Vivian B. Brown and Chi Hughes are affiliated with PROTO-TYPES, Culver City, CA. A. T. Panter is affiliated with the University of North Carolina at Chapel Hill and The Measurement Group.

Address correspondence to: G. J. Huba, PhD, The Measurement Group, 5811A Uplander Way, Culver City, CA 90230 (E-mail: ghuba@TheMeasurementGroup. com).

This work was supported in part by the Health Resources and Services Administration (HRSA), HIV/AIDS Bureau (HAB), Special Projects of National Significance (SPNS) Grant No. 5 U90 HA 00030-05. This publication's contents are solely the responsibility of the authors and do not necessarily represent the official view of the funding agency.

[Haworth co-indexing entry note]: "Conceptual Issues in Implementing and Using Evaluation in the 'Real World' Setting of a Community-Based Organization for HIV/AIDS Services." Huba, G. J. et al. Co-published simultaneously in *Drugs & Society* (The Haworth Press, Inc.) Vol. 16, No. 1/2, 2000, pp. 31-54; and: *Evaluating HIV/AIDS Treatment Programs: Innovative Methods and Findings* (ed: G. J. Huba et al.) The Haworth Press, Inc., 2000, pp. 31-54. Single or multiple copies of this article are available for a fee from The Haworth Document Delivery Service [1-800-342-9678, 9:00 a.m. - 5:00 p.m. (EST). E-mail address: getinfo@haworthpressinc.com].

tion must accommodate to one another. Examples of the interplay of the first two issues and their resolution are given. *[Article copies available for a fee from The Haworth Document Delivery Service: 1-800-342-9678. E-mail address: <getinfo@haworthpressinc.com> Website: <http://www.HaworthPress. com>]*

KEYWORDS. Evaluation, CBO, real world

INTRODUCTION

In the past several decades, Community-Based Organizations, or CBOs, have often acted as a natural "laboratory" or "testing ground" for innovative services and service models, especially for groups of individuals who are disenfranchised within society and from the traditional institutions that provide medical, social, and other needed human services (e.g., Hammett, Gaiter, & Crawford, 1998; LeBlanc, 1997). The importance of CBOs as places where new programs can be implemented, tested, and nurtured, has been well-illustrated in the case of HIV/AIDS services. When AIDS was first detected, newly-formed CBOs were able to design responsive treatment systems that could attract those individuals most likely to be affected by the disease into potentially needed medical treatment and social services. The CBOs recognized that unlike other existing human service organizations, those individuals likely to be affected by HIV were disenfranchised from traditional institutions because of their sexual orientation, status as an ethnic-racial minority, gender, substance abuse, and lack of health insurance. That is, CBOs recognized early in the HIV epidemic that the groups at highest risk to contract HIV would potentially be under-utilizers of traditional services (Huba & Melchior, 1994; Weissman, Melchior, Huba, Altice, Booth, Cottler, Genser, Jones, McCarthy, Needle, & Smereck, 1995; Weissman & Brown, 1996).

Among the services emphasized by the HIV/AIDS CBO movement were those tailored to the special needs of the client, those encouraging clients to be a "partner" in their own treatment, and those eliminating structural and social barriers to accessing services. The CBO movement has also historically been quite important in the development of innovative substance abuse, mental health, and community medical services, especially for those individuals traditionally under-served. Because CBOs have been responsive to the service needs of their clients and developed innovative service models, many have been selected as "national demonstration projects" by various federal and local funding agencies.

A key part of innovating services is to develop clinical models that can be evaluated for their effectiveness. As part of their national demonstration project funding, many CBOs are currently receiving funds that permit them to design and implement evaluations of their service effectiveness and outcomes. As these evaluations are developed, it is important that the unique characteristics of CBOs that make them such important sources of service innovation be captured in evaluations that show the program strengths rather than forcing them into traditional designs that may be more appropriate for traditional services following a "clinical trials" model. It is our contention that more traditional, experimental design-based evaluations, although rigorous in a textbook sense, may "miss" some of the truly unique, effective, and innovative aspects of a CBO model. Consequently, in this paper we discuss the potentially competing issues that arise from programmatic considerations and rigorous evaluation design considerations. We suggest various "hybrid" and blended evaluation techniques–not necessarily following traditional experimental designs–that may be most effective for capturing the true outcomes of the CBO programs. It is the major point of this paper to highlight that when such considerations conflict, the ability of the program to deliver the most effective services must be maximized in a way most appropriate for its clients even if it entails using a non-traditional, perhaps less rigorous, evaluation design that blends elements from many possible kinds of studies.

There are three sections that follow in this paper. In the first section, we discuss some unique programmatic considerations of CBOs that must be considered in designing and implementing an effective evaluation. In the second section, we discuss some major evaluation design issues that must be resolved to design a valid evaluation. In the third section, we discuss how the program may accommodate slightly to the evaluation considerations and the evaluation may accommodate greatly to the programmatic considerations.

A Model for Understanding Programmatic and Evaluation Considerations and Their Intersection

In Sections 1 and 2, we discuss 10 programmatic and evaluation considerations. In each of these sections we differentiate Level I, Level II, and Level III issues. Generally speaking, Level I concerns are very broad global ones that mainly impact the program and the evaluator in very general ways that are not specific to the program being evaluated. Level II issues are more specific to the local program and the evaluation. Finally, Level III issues are most specific to the program and its evaluation. Both the program and the evaluator must deal with Level I, Level II, and Level III issues. Of the most importance is how issues from different levels intersect. After discussing these issues for the program and the evaluator separately, we will summarize the 10 major issues in terms of the interaction of program and evaluation perspectives.

Section 1: Unique Programmatic Considerations of Community-Based Organizations

As noted, there are a number of unique programmatic considerations in Community-Based Organizations that must be taken into account in the evaluation process. In the examples that follow, we have explicitly used as an example issues faced in a Community-Based Organization that has as its primary mission provision of HIV/AIDS services. It should be noted, however, that there are parallel (and in most cases, virtually identical) issues in other types of CBOs including those with primary missions of providing substance abuse, mental health, or community primary healthcare services.

Table 1 shows 10 major issues in implementing an evaluation within an HIV/AIDS CBO from the program standpoint. There are three clusters of issues discussed here. At the most general level (Level I) for an HIV/AIDS CBO, there must first be an explicit recognition in the program design that the *medical state-of-the-art* for HIV/AIDS treatment is changing rapidly, and that changes continue to happen at a faster pace as medical science advances in the treatment of the disease. Bartlett (1999) discusses the state-of-the-art in such treatments as protease inhibitor combination therapy or highly active anti-retroviral therapy (HAART) and its monitoring with viral load testing. Such new medical therapies lead to an increased understanding of the medical management of HIV, as well as needed social supports to ensure adherence to effective medical treatments. As medical treatments for HIV change rapidly, CBOs must realize that their knowledge of the medical therapies that they recommend and provide supports for will change, often from month-to-month. Constant to this change, however, are a number of non-changing facts: (a) at least some clients will not necessarily understand complicated medical therapies and how to correctly follow physician instructions; (b) clients must be emotionally supported in adhering to their medical therapies; (c) at least some clients will have concomitant emotional and behavioral problems that must be addressed in order for their medical therapies to be effective; and (d) for any new therapy, at least some proportion of the patients will not respond medically and must be helped to move to other potentially effective therapies.

A second general issue for the CBO providing HIV/AIDS services is that the *national context* of HIV/AIDS also is changing. In the earliest phases of the epidemic in the United States, the groups most heavily impacted by HIV were men who have sex with men and hemophiliacs; these groups came from very diverse social-economic backgrounds and were not clustered in the poorest brackets. At the next wave of the epidemic, injection drug users and their sex partners were impacted heavily and joined the treatment populations. In later phases of the epidemic, women, youth, people of color, individuals at the lowest SES brackets, and crack drug users have become disproportionately impacted by the disease. At the same time, there have been shifts in social and medical programs such as changing eligibility standards for those programs–Medicaid, Welfare–that traditionally supported individuals who are either without resources for medical treatment or who exhaust such re-

TABLE 1. Major Considerations of a Community-Based Organization Participating in a Demonstration Project (Example: HIV/AIDS Services)

Level I: Broad and Theoretical/Contextual

1. *Changes in Treatment State-of-the-Art:* Medical and psychosocial treatment standards change rapidly

   - Protease inhibitor treatment/HAART therapy
   - Viral load testing
   - Continuously evolving more sophisticated understanding of medical management of HIV
   - Changing models for case management and social supports
   - Models for treating psychosocial and medical co-morbidities

2. *National Context for HIV Disease*

   - Changing epidemiology of HIV/AIDS and groups most affected
   - Welfare reform and expected financial resources of treatment populations
   - Managed care

3. *Multiple Funding Streams*

   - Different funders (federal, state, local) will each pay for specific services within an overall program each wants to manage
   - Co-mingling, leveraging, and continuity of funding sources

Level II: More Specific and Local

4. *Local Context for HIV Service Delivery*

   - What the local county is paying for, Title I politics, HIV consortium, and local priority setting
   - Continuity of local treatment models and funding streams in response to shifting state-of-the-art and directed federal/state funding

5. *Matching Program Staff to Target Clients*

   - Recruitment and retention of <u>staff</u> and <u>clients</u> in a CBO while trying to be sensitive to people with HIV
   - Wanting to have staff who are living with HIV but need to worry about issues like training, relapse, special schedules

6. *Termination of Treatment/Program Length*

   - Traditional idea is to have people get the services they need and leave but since HIV is a chronic disease it requires modification of traditional time- and resource-limited CBO models
   - Retention of sick and "distressed" clients in the program
   - Co-managed versus solely-managed clients
   - Integrated versus parallel services
   - Perceived relative importance–by different constituency groups–of psychosocial (CBO) as opposed to medical (pharmaceutical, managed care) services

Level III: Very Specific and Central

7. *Designing Program Under Grant Initiative*

   - Balancing the original RFP terms, the reality of implementation, the national direction of HIV/AIDS services and funding, current state-of-the-art

8. *Sustainability*

   - Increase expectation in the community that services will be there forever, when in reality there are only 3-5 years of "augmented" demonstration funding available
   - Agency feels responsible for sustaining a needed and successful program
   - Agency will start to change the program almost from the beginning to ensure additional, sustained funding from other sources
   - Funders are generally unwilling to allow original program to replicate its results with alternate populations, in other locales, and in other contexts

9. *Services for Underserved, Affected Populations*

   - Services need to be appropriate and sensitive to the target population
   - Multiple-disenfranchisements in services: ethnicity, sexual orientation, gender, co-morbidities, financial
   - Use medical and psychosocial models designed specifically for original target population

10. *Program Treatment Model*

    - Treatment Model has to flow from the Agency Model
    - As the state-of-the-art changes [Issues 1-9] how does the Treatment Model change?
    - Practical implementation to provide maximally effective services under the Agency and Treatment Models

sources and cannot work. Simultaneously, new economic models for medical services through managed care and privatization have changed the way that individuals in publicly-supported programs receive their care. CBOs in the HIV/AIDS field must be responsive to such changes, many of which occur in short periods of time and impact a high percentage of the client population.

As the national context for HIV services has changed at the same time the number of individuals impacted by the disease has increased, a number of fractionated programs have been funded nationally and locally. These programs create a context in which a typical disenfranchised, sick, and poor client of a CBO may obtain housing services paid for by one federal or local agency, medical services paid for by another federal or local agency, psycho-social services paid for by a third federal or local agency, and case management paid for by a fourth federal or local agency designed to ensure that this confused state somehow comes together. CBOs thus face issues of continuity of funding from various sources that may give them resources for "partial" programs for a limited time. Within such co-mingling of resources, it is potentially difficult to disentangle the effects of one kind of funding as opposed to another as part of the salary of a case manager may be paid for by one funding source while another funding source pays the remainder of her salary *to serve the same clients.*

At a second level (Level II) for CBOs are more immediate local issues. Among these, there is first the issue of local context which supplements national context. At the local level, for HIV there may be a (Title I) planning council, funding from the County or City, and local advisory boards or consortia. These local groups may have many of the same dynamics as the national context and may change their priorities just as rapidly, or even more so. A second Level II issue is that potential programmatic discontinuity might occur because of issues in the retention of staff and clients within the CBO. A successful CBO often incorporates in its staff individuals who themselves are consumers of services of the type offered by the program. For instance, an HIV/AIDS CBO may have one or more key staff members who potentially can be ill for a period of time from HIV or have some other problem (such as relapsing to substance abuse) with a resulting discontinuity in staffing or client recruitment. A third Level II issue for the CBO, and especially in the HIV/AIDS area, is that the concept of "termination" of treatment or services has been changed. In the case of HIV/AIDS, the virus represents a chronic disease; in the case of substance abuse or mental illness there is generally a need for continuing support services; in the case of a community health clinic there is need to keep the client returning for primary health services. Client retention is a key goal. Because clients will potentially be staying in services indefinitely, their service episodes are not simple ones and in fact during a service episode there may be a shift in what is provided, who provides it, who funds the services, and how integrated the services themselves are.

At the level of the specific treatment model implemented by the CBO, there are a number of Level III issues which most directly impact upon what is going to happen within the CBO on a day-to-day basis. The first of these issues is a *balancing* of three considerations: (a) what was the project funded to do? (b) what can the project actually do with the money when it sits down to hire staff and design a program? and (c) how does the national-local context for the services at the time they are implemented push the program in one direction or another? A second Level III issue is one that might be called *program sustainability.* Programs that are started and enroll clients need to be designed in such a way that they can continue even if the original funding source is not present. Program design to ensure sustainability may include shifts from the original plan as new (co-) funding streams are added to the program or economies of scale and design are implemented. An unfortunate consequence of the national context for demonstration programs is that their demonstration funding is explicitly limited (usually to fairly short periods of 3-5 years), and accordingly most programs will need to start looking for sustaining funding, and implement changes required by new funders, almost from the start of their initial funding.

Another Level III program issue is that of developing services that are appropriate for, and sensitive to, *specific populations.* Consider the example of women seeking services for HIV/AIDS. Older medical and social models of treatment for HIV–derived for populations of men who have sex with men–may not fit the needs of women. Medical models derived in clinical trials often did not include women, and if they did, generally limited themselves to issues of physiological responsiveness, rather than total responsiveness to the regimen. Because the populations for new medical treatments have traditionally been homogeneous, those groups not included in the original trials are at a disadvantage for state-of-the-art treatments. A key issue for CBOs has been to adapt state-of-the-art treatments to additional populations, many of whom have needs that are somewhat different from those of the original groups studied. What this means from a pragmatic viewpoint is that CBOs will usually have programs that start with a standard of care that was defined for another population then add some experimental elements to "proven" treatments in order to make them appropriate and sensitive to under-represented groups.

The final Level III issue lies at the core of the CBO program and is that of the *Treatment Model* for the program. The Treatment Model is a combination of all of the issues discussed above, drawing most heavily from Level III, and then from Level II and Level I concerns. As the issues in Levels I, II, and III change, the Treatment Model of the program often will change. The Treatment Model for the program must also be understood within the overall model for the agency in which the program exists. The larger agency–of which the program may be but a small part–may itself be subject to all of the issues discussed above for the specific program.

Section 2: Unique Considerations Evaluators Bring into Community-Based Organizations

As we have just seen, Community-Based Organizations, typified by the HIV/AIDS CBO, bring various considerations into a national demonstration project that must be considered in the evaluation. Much as CBOs have a purpose, a mission, and a constituency, evaluators also come into the projects with a purpose, a mission, and a constituency. We next turn our attention to 10 issues that evaluators of service demonstration programs may bring into the process. As with the issues that we have just discussed for Community Based Organizations, these considerations are discussed as Level I, II, or III ones depending upon their centrality to a specific evaluation. Table 2 summarizes these issues.

There are several general, or Level I issues that guide the evaluation team as they approach the CBO program and try to develop a valid and fair evaluation. The most general of these issues is the collected set of standards and principles that might be termed *generally-accepted practices for research designs to show the effects of programs.* There are voluminous literatures, covering more than 50 years and thousands of research articles on the advantages and pitfalls of using different kinds of "research or evaluation designs" to study the effects of a program. Collectively the wisdom on balancing a number of competing technical issues might be termed the *practice standards for an evaluation design.* Such standards usually include such issues as treating program participants ethically, using a design that is as objective and reproducible as possible, and one which minimizes the biases of either the evaluator or the program staff that might affect the outcome of the evaluation study. A second general issue is one that might be termed *generally-accepted standards for data collection.* Again, as with the evaluation design, there is voluminous scientific literature on how to measure key variables in a program being evaluated. The evaluation team will be seeking to implement data measurement methods that are reliable in that they can be reproduced by different data collectors at a different time, valid in that they measure what they purport to measure, have fidelity in that they are true measures of program performance, and complete. At this most general level, there is also a third issue that the evaluators will want to consider, and this is the possible federal (or other funding source) context for the type of program that they are trying to evaluate. Specifically, what does the funding or regulatory agency expect that evaluation to show? Is the evaluation part of a general initiative with a cross-cutting or multi-site evaluation?

TABLE 2. Major Considerations of an Evaluator Participating in a Demonstration Project

Level I: Broad and Theoretical/Contextual

1. *Generally-Accepted Research Design Standards*
   - Design sensitive enough to show program effects
2. *Generally-Accepted Data Collection Standards*
   - Reliability, validity, fidelity, and completeness
3. *Federal Context for HIV/AIDS Studies*
   - Local evaluation and its conformity to the national (cross-cutting) evaluation

Level II: More Specific and Local

4. *Evaluator Strengths and Philosophy*
   - Psychologists, Anthropologists, Sociologists, Epidemiologists, Biostatisticians, and professionals from other disciplines
   - Quantitative or qualitative approach
   - Who does the evaluator perceive as the client for the evaluation, the Agency or the Funder?

5. *Generalizable Prior Evaluation Tools*
   - Types of evaluation expertise and prior experiences from the agency and/or the evaluation team
   - Existing tools, and methods that can be adapted
   - Prior work with Community-Based Organizations
   - Prior work with federal or state funding agencies

6. *Development of Sensitive Client-Specific Procedures* as opposed to a generalized approach on instruments and designs
   - Mix of methods appropriate for agency, such as focus groups, data collection methods that are part of clinical services, different things for different kinds of people
   - Sensitivity to staff issues such as staff not collecting data and the necessity of retraining staff periodically after turnover
   - Cultural sensitivity to the population(s) served by the agency and the potential inappropriateness of standardized measures

Level III: Very Specific and Central

7. *Grant Initiative Terms*
   - Design you originally proposed versus what you want to implement and the program that is now being implemented
   - When responding to the Request for Applications, did not know the design of the cross-cutting evaluation for the overall grant initiative or if the program would have to be changed to match an external consensus criterion
   - Don't know how the program will change over time

8. *Sustainability of Evaluation Methods for Agency*
   - Database, MIS systems for agency, help the program get more grants
   - Sustainability of the evaluators (continuing evaluator contracts)
   - Helping evaluate other sources of funding not part of the project (cross-use of data)

9. *Appreciation of Complex Program Model*
   - Design, instruments, sample, procedures (quantitative versus qualitative) to be able to answer many stated and unstated (emergent) questions by the funding agency and the program
   - Sensitivity issues to the program
   - Detect any anomalies in the program
   - Entry point of the evaluator into the process (at program design/grant proposal versus after funding is secured)

10. *Use of Evaluation Information/Results*
    - What gets disseminated
    - Who sees the information disseminated
    - How information is used by staff to improve the program
    - What has to go back to the funding agency and what is optional
    - Who owns the database of all the information collected from the program
    - Sustainability of the data collection and reporting methods

At a more central level to the evaluation, designated as Level II, there are several issues. First, what are the strengths and philosophies of the evaluators? Some evaluation teams tend to favor quantitative methods over qualitative methods, others favor qualitative methods, and still others tend to blend both kinds of methods. The primary professional background of the evaluation team might include many disciplines; some common ones among those evaluators who work with CBOs are the disciplines of psychology, sociology, and public health. In understanding the evaluation approach it is important to consider how the disciplinary background of the evaluators is related to the general service area of the program. Next, how willing are the evaluators to develop sensitive client-specific procedures? Community-Based Organizations often serve clients who have been traditionally underserved, oftentimes using staff drawn from the same groups as the clients. Because CBOs treat a diverse group of individuals, it. is absolutely critical that the evaluator be familiar with assessing individuals who have a limited education, do not speak English as their primary language, are not used to self-completed forms or research interviews, and who tend to view all data collection as a "test" that has to be passed in order to ensure continued access to needed services.

At the most central level to the evaluation of the specific program (Level III), the following issues are important: First, what are the terms of the grant initiative? Are the conditions in the grant initiative actually applicable to the program that the agency has been funded to conduct? Will the overall shape of what was initially proposed have to be changed because of the conditions of the award including requirements from a multi-site evaluation? Second, how can an evaluation be implemented that permits the agency to become more self-sustaining by generating data that allow for continuing quality improvement and the ability to write new grants? Data used for evaluations may also be data used to justify the continuing existence of the agency, or at least to point out unmet needs among the clients the agency serves. Third, how can the evaluator capture the complexity of the program model, its strengths, its trade-offs, and the ways in which staff and clients make decisions about treatment protocols for individual clients? Finally, how does the evaluator intend to communicate the results from the evaluation and to whom will she disseminate the results? Program results are a valuable commodity that can be used to further the program and its sustainability as well as the future career of the evaluator. The results generated and the way in which they are disseminated need to recognize the competing uses for the results and their overall value to all parties.

Section 3: The Intersection of Program and Evaluation Concerns: How the Program May Accommodate to the Evaluation and the Evaluation May Accommodate to the Program

The program and the evaluator each approach their mutual working relationship with the same goal in mind: both want to do the best job possible. As we have just seen, both the program and evaluator tend to bring a set of professional objectives to the working relationship, some of which, if thought of in a rigid way, may be in conflict with one another. It is our argument if the professional objectives of the program and the professional objectives of the evaluator are reconciled in a flexible way, that the program will gain a potentially valuable tool for its own self improvement, while the evaluator will learn new ways of documenting successes which leads to a continuing process of self-improvement for the evaluation team.

As we noted, Table 3 summarizes for the 10 major issues discussed above for the program and the 10 major evaluation issues. Together the intersections of these 10 issues create 100 "cells" where the concerns of the program and those of the evaluation *might* need to be reconciled. Recognizing that both major parties to the evaluation–the program being evaluated and the independent professional interpreting the evaluation–will have certain peripheral and core concerns that need to be explicitly addressed as the evaluation is planned and implemented goes a long way toward avoiding potential conflict through discussion.

Not all of the cells defined by the grid in Table 3 are equally likely to produce a set of conflicts. In the following sections we have picked some of the cells defined by the concerns of the program and those of the evaluator, and we discuss some of the ways that these can be reconciled.

Possible Friction Point 1: "The Data-Staff Crunch." The evaluation will generally be seen as needing as much data as possible while the program staff feels that staff need to devote their own time to serving clients (and *not* collecting data) and the clients need to devote as much of their own time as possible to working on therapeutic objectives (and *not* generating data). How can these objectives be blended together? First, staff can help the evaluator identify both the ongoing data collection that is already done by the program to satisfy funders or to obtain information necessary for assessing client needs or treatment planning. Often, these data will speak directly to at least some of the evaluation objectives and can either be incorporated directly into the evaluation or adapted slightly to meet both needs. Second, as the evaluator looks at ongoing information collection techniques in the agency, it may be possible to design forms or other data entry or data reporting methods for the staff that actually make existing staff tasks easier. For instance, if services need to be tabulated monthly for a funding agency to collect contract reimbursements, the evaluator may be able to collect this information in an easier way, conduct a statistical analysis, and provide the program management with the information thus saving them significant time. Among the techniques that make it easier for staff to collect ongoing data, or new ones, are scannable paper forms that can collect data in a way that is close to existing paper forms used by funding agencies or the program (Huba, Brown &

TABLE 3. Key Questions to Ask About an Evaluation Within the Intersection of Concerns of the Program and the Evaluator

EVALUATION (→) / PROGRAM (↓)	A. Generally Accepted Research Design Standards	B. Generally Accepted Data Collection Standards	C. Federal Context for HIV/AIDS Studies	D. Evaluator Strengths and Philosophy	E. Generalizable Prior Evaluation Tools	F. Development of Sensitive Client-Specific Procedures	G. Grant Initiative Terms	H. Sustainability of Evaluation Methods for Agency	I. Appreciation of Complex Program Model	J. Use of Evaluation Information/Results
1. Changes in Treatment State-of-the-Art	Will the evaluation design allow for probable changes in the program treatment methods?	Will data collection be static through the project, or will new data collection be added as the state-of-the-art treatment program changes?	Do the design and data answer important, new policy questions about HIV/AIDS treatment?	Will the evaluator flexibly respond to changes in the treatment state-of-the-art that require modifications in the program and hence the evaluation design and instruments?	Does the evaluator have access to existing valid tools that permit the assessment of outcomes under differing treatment protocols?	Is the evaluator aware of changes in state-of-the-art treatment that occur during the course of the program?	Are the grant initiative terms sufficiently flexible to allow for changes that may occur during the funding period?	Do the proposed evaluation methods adequately capture state-of-the-art shifts and how the program is dealing with these changes?	Is there an appreciation of the complexity of the program model, especially as it deals with a changing state-of-the-art in HIV care?	Will the evaluation data and findings be reported and disseminated in a way that adequately reflects the changing landscape in treatment state-of-the-art?
2. National Context for HIV Disease	Will the evaluation design allow for possible changes in target populations [and their issues] over time?	Will data collection allow for possible changes in key issues and target populations over time?	Do the design and data inform public policy on the treatment of HIV/AIDS?	Will the evaluator flexibly respond to changes in treatment populations that require modifications in the program and hence the evaluation design and instruments?	Does the evaluator have access to existing valid tools that permit the assessment of outcomes for changing treatment populations?	Is the evaluator aware of the ways that changing treatment populations may change the require-ments for measures and indicators in different years of the program? Will the norms for the measures be adjusted to reflect changing populations over time?	Are the grant initiative terms sufficiently flexible to allow for changes that may occur nationally during the funding period?	Do the proposed evaluation methods adequately capture the national HIV context and how the program interacts within this context?	Is there an appreciation of the complexity of the program model, especially in responding to the national context of HIV disease?	Will the evaluation data and findings be reported and disseminated in a way that adequately addresses the national context for HIV disease?

3. Multiple Funding Streams	Will the evaluation design cover only specific services funded by one initiative, or overall program services? Can the design separate the effects of different funding sources?	Will data collection be useful not only for the specific funding agency for this project but also for other funding sources for the agency?	Do the design and data address issues of co-mingling funds, leveraging resources, and continuity of funding?	Will the evaluator understand the complexity of flexible funding streams in an agency and attempt to incorporate this into the evaluation design?	Does the evaluator have access to existing valid tools that will permit the assessment of outcomes in a way that answers the questions of different funders?	Is the evaluator aware that clients and staff tend to perceive a program as "unitary" and that to pull its parts into separate pieces for evaluation purposes may hinder global treatment efforts?	Are the grant initiative terms sufficiently flexible to allow for simultaneous funding streams that typically sustain a project?	Do the proposed evaluation methods adequately meet the demands required of a multiple funding stream context?	Is there an appreciation of the complexity of the program model, especially as it navigates and balances the demands arising from multiple funding streams?	Will the evaluation data and findings be reported and disseminated in a way that recognizes that the demands of multiple funding streams constrained the evaluation?
4. Local Context for HIV Service Delivery	Will the evaluation design be able to disentangle desired initiative (federal) outcomes from desired local outcomes?	Will data collection document both grant initiative and local issues and outcomes?	Do the evaluation design and data inform public policy on local priority setting processes for the treatment of HIV/AIDS?	Will the evaluator understand the local context of the HIV service system and attempt to also answer key local questions of outcomes and priorities?	Does the evaluator have access to existing valid tools that will permit the assessment of outcomes in a way that informs the local HIV service delivery system?	Is the evaluator aware of changes in the local HIV service delivery system during the course of the program?	Are the grant initiative terms sufficiently flexible to recognize the local context for HIV service delivery?	Do the proposed evaluation methods adequately address the local HIV service delivery system and how the program functions within this system?	Is there an appreciation of the complexity of the program model, especially as it exists in the local HIV service system?	Will the evaluation data and findings be reported and disseminated in a way that adequately addresses the local HIV service delivery system?

TABLE 3 (continued)

EVALUATION (→) PROGRAM (↓)	A. Generally Accepted Research Design Standards	B. Generally Accepted Data Collection Standards	C. Federal Context for HIV/AIDS Studies	D. Evaluator Strengths and Philosophy	E. Generalizable Prior Evaluation Tools	F. Development of Sensitive Client-Specific Procedures	G. Grant Initiative Terms	H. Sustainability of Evaluation Methods for Agency	I. Appreciation of Complex Program Model	J. Use of Evaluation Information/ Results
5. Matching Program Staff to Target Clients	Will the evaluation design be able to examine the effects of the similarity of clients and staff?	Will data collection methods and tools be appropriate both for the target clients and for the skill levels of the staff expected to collect the information?	Do the design and data inform public policy on the importance of matching staff and client attributes?	Will the evaluator be able to design methods and procedures appropriate to both the target client population and the staff expected to collect the information? Does the evaluator have the sensitivity to empower staff and clients to critique the design and tools and collect information?	Does the evaluator have access to existing valid tools that will permit the assessment of outcomes for diverse treatment populations served by staff from differing professional and cultural backgrounds?	Is the evaluator aware of the similarity between staff and clients in designing data collection procedures?	Are the grant initiative terms sufficiently flexible to reflect the program reality in which program staff is well matched to target clients?	Do the proposed evaluation methods adequately capture the importance of matching program staff with client attributes?	Is there an appreciation of the complexity of the program model, especially as it seeks to match program staff and client attributes?	Will the evaluation data and findings be reported and disseminated in a way that adequately reflects the importance of matching program staff to client attributes?

6. Termination of Treatment/ Program Length	Will the evaluation design be able to document both inter-vention specific outcomes and out-comes from long-term chronic client man-agement? Can data be collected from outside service providers that the client encounters during an overall treatment episode (e.g., emergency rooms, specialty care providers)?	Are data collection methods appropriate at different levels of overall disease level (functioning) and for repeated assessments during a long-term treatment episode?	Do the design and data inform public policy on the importance of long-term continuing care as opposed to alternate managed care models?	Is the evaluator able to address technical issues that arise from real-world treatment episodes in which clients may or may not choose to receive services and to complete data collection procedures?	Does the evaluator have access to existing valid tools that work well in real-world treatment episodes in which clients may or may not choose to receive services and to complete data collection procedures?	Is the evaluator aware of how to capture the different reasons why changes in program status may occur and other issues of program retention?	Are the grant initiative terms sufficiently flexible to allow for all situations that might lead a client to terminate services or choose to have a discontinuous pattern of treatment and services?	Do the proposed evaluation methods adequately capture how clients move in and out of services?	Is there an appreciation of the complexity of the program model, especially as it attempts to track all patterns of service use?	Will the evaluation data and findings be reported and disseminated in a way that adequately reflects differential patterns of retention and the complex reasons for disruption of services for some clients?

TABLE 3 (continued)

EVALUATION (→) PROGRAM (↓)	A. Generally Accepted Research Design Standards	B. Generally Accepted Data Collection Standards	C. Federal Context for HIV/AIDS Studies	D. Evaluator Strengths and Philosophy	E. Generalizable Prior Evaluation Tools	F. Development of Sensitive Client-Specific Procedures	G. Grant Initiative Terms	H. Sustainability of Evaluation Methods for Agency	I. Appreciation of Complex Program Model	J. Use of Evaluation Information/Results
7. Designing Program Under Grant Initiative	Will the evaluation design answer the questions raised in the grant initiative?	Are data collection methods appropriate to answer the questions raised in the grant initiative?	Do the design and data permit a valid assessment of the effects and outcomes of the program as it was implemented and conducted throughout the entire funding period?	Is the evaluator able to document and understand the trade-offs that occur from meeting the mandates of multiple funding streams and to document the program "as implemented" as opposed to "as designed?"	Does the evaluator have access to existing valid tools that permit the assessment of outcomes that reflect grant initiative goals as well as implemented design goals?	Is the evaluator aware of the need to design procedures that both address aspects of the specific "proposed" program under the grant initiative and the "as implemented" version of the program?	Are the grant initiative terms sufficiently flexible to allow for the inevitable discrepancies between the proposed program and the implemented one?	Do the proposed evaluation methods reflect the current implemented program?	Is there an appreciation of the complexity of the program model, especially as it reconciles proposed designs with the realities of implementing the program?	Will the evaluation data and findings be reported and disseminated in a way that adequately reflects the demands of implementing the original proposed work versus the reality and design shifts due to the actual treatment and program context?

8. Sustainability	Are the data collected appropriate to allow the agency to apply for additional follow-on funding from the same or additional sources?	Do the design and data permit an assessment by funding sources about the importance of sustaining or replicating the model?	Is the evaluator sensitive to the ways in which evaluation results may be used to determine which program components to maintain through follow-on funding? Is the evaluator aware of how evaluation results and data may be used to justify the program for future funding?	Does the evaluator have access to existing valid tools that permit an assessment of outcomes that will permit the agency to "make the case" for continued funding?	Is the evaluator aware of designing procedures that can maximize the probability that the program will be reflective positively for subsequent funding initiatives?	Are the grant initiative terms sufficiently flexible to allow for needed additional data collection efforts to insure that a program has shown success and is therefore sustainable?	Do the proposed evaluation methods adequately capture the importance of insuring that the program will be sustained and replicated in the future?	Is there an appreciation of the complexity of the program model, especially as it attempts to insure its sustainability while still offering the highest possible HIV care to clients?	Will the evaluation data and findings be reported and disseminated in a way that shows the program in the best light it can be and not blur findings in a way that can jeopardize subsequent funding?
Does the evaluation design leave skills and methods in the agency that can be maintained after the end of the specific grant? Does the evaluation design help identify program components that should be separately sustained even if the entire program cannot be maintained?									

TABLE 3 (continued)

EVALUATION (→) / PROGRAM (↓)	A. Generally Accepted Research Design Standards	B. Generally Accepted Data Collection Standards	C. Federal Context for HIV/AIDS Studies	D. Evaluator Strengths and Philosophy	E. Generalizable Prior Evaluation Tools	F. Development of Sensitive Client-Specific Procedures	G. Grant Initiative Terms	H. Sustainability of Evaluation Methods for Agency	I. Appreciation of Complex Program Model	J. Use of Evaluation Information/Results
9. Services for Underserved	Is the evaluation design appropriate and sensitive for all individuals likely to be served by the program?	Are the instruments and tools appropriate and sensitive for all individuals likely to be served by the program?	Do the design and data inform public policy about accessibility and inclusion of high-need populations?	Is the evaluator sensitive to the complex issues of the valid interpretation of outcomes for diverse treatment populations and aware that a specific outcome may have different implications for different groups?	Does the evaluator have access to existing valid tools that permit the assessment of service patterns for underserved clients?	Is the evaluator aware of designing procedures that will adequately capture how underserved clients enter and engage in services?	Are the grant initiative terms sufficiently flexible to allow for provision of services for underserved clients?	Do the proposed evaluation methods adequately demonstrate the need to link underserved clients to services?	Is there an appreciation of the complexity of the program model, especially as it continues to insure that underserved clients receive services?	Will the evaluation data and findings be reported and disseminated in a way that adequately captures the importance of providing services to the underserved?

10. Program Treatment Model	Does the evaluation design fully take into account the complexity and richness of the program model without requiring a change in the model to accommodate the evaluation design?	Do the instruments and tools permit a full and accurate portrayal of the program model and its outcomes?	Do the design and data permit the funding agency to validly and unequivocally determine the success of the program model?	Is the evaluator able to understand the full richness and complexity of a program model as it evolves over time to meet the changing needs of diverse treatment populations?	Does the evaluator have access to existing valid tools that permit the assessment of outcomes that are specific to unique aspects of the program treatment model?	Is the evaluator aware of designing procedures that do not interfere with a changing and dynamic program treatment model?	Are the grant initiative terms sufficiently flexible to allow a program model that necessarily will shift to reflect the current, more beneficial set of treatments, as noted by program staff during the course of the funding period?	Do the proposed evaluation methods adequately capture the full complexity of the program model?	Is there an appreciation of the complexity of the program model, especially as it attempts to be true to its original missions and goals?	Will the evaluation data and findings be reported and disseminated in a way that captures the richness and complexity of the particular program model?

Melchior, 1995). Such forms have been shown to be useful by groups ranging from street outreach workers to professional staff; the training required to collect data in this way is minimal if the forms are close to the ongoing reporting requirements for the program. Third, the evaluator can help the program staff identify ways to use new data collection tools to better serve the client by identifying her needs more accurately, helping to show intermediate outcomes or progress, and document ongoing areas needing further work. That is, new data collection methods introduced to show overall program outcomes may be quite useful as tools for staff to use in assessing individual client progress and outcomes.

Possible Friction Point 2: "I don't want to show you what I know how to do so you can't do it." Evaluators tend to live and die by the quality of data they have available and the way that the data are collected in adherence to a formal design. In doing so, and in asking program staff to collect data that are required on designated days, there may be a tendency by the evaluation staff to consider the program staff as "data collectors" who need not know how the data collection methods were designed and what possible theoretical problems of interpretation and validity the evaluation design will address. Program staff deal on a daily basis with the ongoing and changing needs of clients and the ways that these needs can be met within changing program staffing, changing program levels of funding, and changing linked service networks with differing levels of opportunity for outside referrals for client needs that are beyond the scope of the program. As the program dynamically changes and the client population changes, program staff may consider these changes to be "clinical issues" that are not very important for the evaluators to know about, or they may observe that the evaluation no longer seems relevant to the way that the program works, perhaps attributing this to a lack of interest on the part of the evaluators about these clinical or programmatic issues. Evaluators may be prone to concluding that the clinical staff are not interested in evaluation issues, motivated to learn about them, or possess the requisite technical skills to understand the techniques. Clinical staff may be prone to concluding that the evaluation staff are not interested in clinical issues, motivated to learn about them, or possess the requisite clinical skills to understand the techniques. Getting around such perceptions is a key to both a successful evaluation and to continuing development of both program and evaluation staff; to do so tends to require significant commitment to this by both senior program management and the senior evaluators.

Some advantages of making the development of evaluation skills a priority among the clinical staff are: (a) program staff learn how "objective" or "outside" observers come up with questions about how the program works and the ways in which it can demonstrate effectiveness; (b) program staff learn how data can be generated or collected that allow them to capture those outcomes and events that demonstrate programmatic successes; (c) staff learn how ongoing data collection can provide feedback necessary to improve program quality as well as outcomes for individual clients; (d) staff learn how to collect information that will allow them to justify expanding the program by offering other needed services; (e) program staff can learn how some of the standard ways of conducting evaluations are not clinically sensitive to clients and can help the evaluators design more appropriate procedures; and (f) program staff can help the evaluation staff identify gaps in the evaluation design occurring because the data collection methods or design are not sensitive to important program outcomes. Advantages of making the development of program (or clinical) skills a priority among the evaluation staff include: (a) evaluation staff learn how to understand the ongoing treatment protocols for clients; (b) within the context of the treatment protocols, individual client treatment plans, and program goals, the evaluation staff can come to view program success for individual clients in a broader way wherein "success" is a continuous process and not a simple outcome captured by a few data indicators; (c) evaluation staff can learn the importance of treatment team approaches that stress the synergistic effects of different kinds of services for different kinds of clients; (d) evaluation staff can learn about the burdens of data collection for the clients and the program staff and potentially reduce the load by eliminating redundant or secondary data items; (e) evaluation staff can monitor the validity of the data collection efforts in capturing the client and program successes perceived by the clients and program staff; and (f) evaluation staff can help the clinical staff understand the general patterns of services in the program including possible treatment gaps, emerging client needs, or unanticipated outcomes.

Possible Friction Point 3: "It's my party (data) and I'll do what I want to; you would cry too if it happened to you." The data that come out of an evaluation have significant consequences for the reputation of the program evaluated, the professional reputations of the program management and staff, and the professional reputations of the evaluation team. The results could have direct or indirect bearing on the ability of the program to obtain continued funding, the salaries of the program staff, and the salaries of the evaluator. And, most importantly, the evaluation data can determine whether treatment opportunities of various kinds continue to be available for current and potential clients in either the same, decreased, or expanded quantities. The potential for data misuse, data under-use, or data over-use decreases directly in proportion to the ability of the evaluation staff and program staff to communicate effectively with one another. In these cases, the data can be reported and interpreted within the proper program and design context, with appropriate caveats about possible data limitations, and most importantly, through relating numerical effects to observable clinical changes.

To an evaluator working alone, a "statistically significant" difference may be sufficient grounds to publish a result in a prestigious, peer-reviewed journal. However, without the judgment of program staff about the clinical significance of the result, the true importance of the finding may be missed. A "seven-point difference" on a 20-point scale or "explaining 18% of the variance" may be extremely important because it means the difference between a reasonably well-functioning individual and one who can not autonomously function, or it may be a relatively minor change. Clinical staff might also be able to point out reasons for the change (or lack thereof) that are not apparent merely from examining the research design. Conversely, a program staff member untrained in evaluation, may tend to over-interpret a "favorable" result based on too small a sample or a design with possible confounding factors. Both types of input are important as data are analyzed and presented outside of the program. If the program and the evaluator have jointly trained program staff well to have evaluation skills and evaluation staff to have an appreciation for clinical skills, then data misuse should not be an issue. If the program and evaluation staff have not had the opportunity to expand their skills throughout the evaluation process, then a formal mechanism needs to be considered. For example, a mechanism may involve having the program staff always review results from the evaluation team before they are presented outside the program with having the evaluation staff having access to program staff to help them explain results they question. It seems to us that it is inappropriate for the evaluation staff to assume that they own the data because it is in their computers and that their interpretations will necessarily be correct.

Possible Friction Point 4, "The clients keep asking me questions" or consumers taught empowerment as part of their programs actually want to understand the evaluation results. Community-based organizations traditionally serve those individuals who are not served by more traditional service models. Such individuals–those with HIV/AIDS, those who abuse drugs, those with mental illness, those too poor to have insurance–need to be taught as part of their program how to access services within the traditional service system. Indeed, the concept of client empowerment is a key element in virtually every successful CBO program. Such empowerment, however, does not stop when the intervention is over. Clients often participate actively in their own treatment programs and treatment planning. Sometimes they become staff of the program after successfully participating in the CBO services. Whether clients are still receiving services or are later providing them, a part of their empowerment is to question why they are being asked evaluation questions, what the data show, and how the data are used to justify their service programs. Evaluators who do not recognize that empowered clients question established and standard procedures are living in a textbook-induced daze.

Possible Friction Point 5: "I say questionnaires, and you say focus groups." In CBO programs, the program needs "hard" numbers to satisfy funders and to both evaluate its programs and justify them through contract compliance audits. Nonetheless, the clients of a CBO program are oftentimes not traditional "research subjects" and in fact their experiences are complicated ones perhaps not captured in standard, "validated" quantitative measures. In such cases qualitative data collection through open-ended questions and focus groups can serve to supplement traditional structured interviews and questionnaires. It should be emphasized that what we are talking about is a combination of qualitative and quantitative methods, rather than the self-limiting debate among evaluators and program staff of whether qualitative versus quantitative methods are "better." Note that program staff can, by their clinical training, be an important part of both qualitative data collection and quantifying clinical judgments.

Possible Friction Point 6: "I want my budget." Program staff want to use every penny of a grant to provide services to the needy and underserved individuals they help every day. Evaluators want to ensure that adequate support are available to ensure that key data are collected, that sound analyses can be conducted, and that the results can be fully disseminated. Often, a number of "about 15% of a total grant budget should go into program evaluation" is bandied about and attributed to "federal agencies." However, as with all general guidelines, such a number can either be more than is necessary or woefully inadequate. To determine the appropriate budget for the evaluation, the expectations of the program, the evaluator, and the funding agency need to be very explicit. Usually, it is most difficult to get the funding agency to commit to realistic objectives for the total budget of the project (that is, the total allocated to services and evaluation). Other important considerations are the evaluation purposes, whether the evaluation substitutes for an ongoing management information system (MIS), the mix of quantitative and qualitative data collection, and whether the project is participating in a multi-site evaluation that overlays significant additional costs. What is an appropriate budget percentage to get a real, interactive, partnership process as opposed to an outside imposition of a design? The answer to this question is not difficult to determine if the agency, funder, and evaluator are really operating as a partnership, and the answer is almost impossible to determine if the agency and evaluator are not working from the same assumptions.

CONCLUSION

A good partnership between a Community-Based Organization and the evaluator of its programs can be of substantial value for the CBO, the evaluator, and the funding agency. The reputations of both the program and the evaluator can be enhanced by a successful partnership and state-of-the-art work. Perhaps the best way to ensure that exceptional work is accomplished by both the program and evaluator is to remember the key reason that both roles exist–to determine the success of programs designed to benefit the most under-served and vulnerable members of the society and then to make the most successful models more widely available to such individuals. Given a shared mission to improve and expand services, there are very few potential conflicts between a highly committed and effective CBO and a highly committed and skilled evaluation team that cannot be readily resolved to the ultimate benefit of the program's clients. The remaining papers in this volume examine evaluations of some successful national demonstration programs on HIV that target substance abusers among their treatment populations. We believe that the papers in this volume illustrate a number of different approaches with the successful implementation of an evaluation within an innovative service program to ensure that clients with HIV/AIDS receive the best possible services.

REFERENCES

Bartlett, J. G. (1999). *Medical Management of HIV Infection.* (1999 Edition). Baltimore, MD: Johns Hopkins University, Dept. of Infection Diseases.

Hammett, T. M., Gaiter, J. L., & Crawford, C. (1998). Reaching seriously at-risk populations: Health interventions in criminal justice settings. *Health Education & Behavior, 25* (1), 99-120.

Huba, G. J., Brown, V. B., & Melchior, L. A. (1995). Fax-in forms as a technology for evaluating community projects: An example of HIV risk reduction. *Educational and Psychological Measurement, 55* (1), 75-83.

Huba, G. J., & Melchior, L. A. (1994). *Evaluation of the Effects of Ryan White Title I Funding on Services for HIV-Infected Drug Abusers: Summary Report & Executive Summary for Year 1: Baseline.* U.S. Dept. of Health and Human Services Pub No. HRSA-RD-SP-94-8. A joint project of the Health Resources and Services Administration, the National Institute on Drug Abuse, and the Consortium on Drug Abuse and HIV Services Access.

LeBlanc. R. G. (1997). Definitions of oppression. *Nursing Inquiry, 4* (4), 257-261.

Weissman, G., & Brown, V. B. (1996). Drug using women and HIV: Access to care and treatment issues. In A. O'Leary & L. S. Jemmott (Eds.), *Women and AIDS: Coping and Care.* (pp. 109-121). New York: Plenum.

Weissman, G., Melchior, L., Huba, G., Altice, F., Booth, R., Cottler, L., Genser, S., Jones, A., McCarthy, S., Needle, R., & Smereck, G. (1995). Women living with substance abuse and HIV disease: Medical care access issues. *Journal of the American Medical Women's Association, 50* (3-4), 115-120.

Lessons Learned
in Reducing Barriers to Care:
Reflections from the Community Perspective

Vivian B. Brown, PhD
Anne Stanton, MSW, CSW
Geoffrey A. D. Smereck, AB, JD
Sandra McDonald
Tracey Gallagher
Eustache Jean-Louis, MD, MPH
Chi Hughes, MSW
J. Wallace Kemp
Michael Kennedy, MS, MFCC
Diana E. Brief, PhD

Vivian B. Brown and Chi Hughes are affiliated with PROTOTYPES, Culver City, CA. Anne Stanton and Michael Kennedy are affiliated with the Larkin Street Youth Center, San Francisco, CA. Geoffrey A. D. Smereck is affiliated with the Well-Being Institute, Ann Arbor, MI. Sandra McDonald and J. Wallace Kemp are affiliated with Outreach, Inc., Atlanta, GA. Tracey Gallagher is associated with The Fortune Society, New York, NY. Eustache Jean-Louis is associated with The Center for Community Health Education and Research, Dorchester, MA. The late Diana E. Brief was affiliated with The Measurement Group, Culver City, CA.

Address correspondence to: Vivian B. Brown, PhD, PROTOTYPES, 5601 West Slauson Avenue, Suite #200, Culver City, CA 90230.

This work was supported in part by the Health Resources and Services Administration (HRSA), HIV/AIDS Bureau (HAB), Special Projects of National Significance (SPNS) Grant No. 5 U90 HA 00030-05 (PROTOTYPES and The Measurement Group), BRU900114-05 (Larkin Street Youth Center), BRU900102-05 (Well-Being Institute), BRU900111-05 (Outreach, Inc.), BRU900107-05 (The Fortune Society), and BRU900123-05 (The Center for Community Health Education and Research). The publication's contents are solely the responsibility of the authors and do not necessarily represent the official view of the funding agency.

[Haworth co-indexing entry note]: "Lessons Learned in Reducing Barriers to Care: Reflections from the Community Perspective." Brown, Vivian B. et al. Co-published simultaneously in *Drugs & Society* (The Haworth Press, Inc.) Vol. 16, No. 1/2, 2000, pp. 55-74; and: *Evaluating HIV/AIDS Treatment Programs: Innovative Methods and Findings* (ed: G. J. Huba et al.) The Haworth Press, Inc., 2000, pp. 55-74. Single or multiple copies of this article are available for a fee from The Haworth Document Delivery Service [1-800-342-9678, 9:00 a.m. - 5:00 p.m. (EST). E-mail address: getinfo@haworthpressinc.com].

SUMMARY. Six projects targeting individuals traditionally under-served by the HIV care system performed a cross-cutting evaluation of their programs. Using qualitative and quantitative techniques, the programs showed that they had enrolled more than 1,400 individuals living with HIV. At intake, the clients cited numerous barriers they had previously encountered in approaching services. The clients had high levels of drug abuse, very few had earned income, and most were members of ethnic-racial minority groups. The strategies used by these projects for recruiting hard-to-reach, traditionally underserved individuals appear to be effective. Issues in designing and implementing projects in community-based organizations are discussed. *[Article copies available for a fee from The Haworth Document Delivery Service: 1-800-342-9678. E-mail address: <getinfo@haworthpressinc.com> Website: <http://www.HaworthPress.com>]*

KEYWORDS. Cross-cutting evaluation, CBO, underserved populations

Through its Special Projects of National Significance (SPNS) funding, the Health Resources and Services Administration (HRSA) HIV/AIDS Bureau (HAB) assists in the development of innovative, validated models for HIV/AIDS care that can be adapted and replicated in a variety of settings. In 1994, HRSA awarded 27 grants to projects that were targeting underserved populations. The 27 projects met quarterly and adapted a cross-cutting evaluation (Huba, Melchior, Hillary, Singer, & Marconi, 1998). Extended descriptions of the projects and their evaluation results are given on the Internet at www.TheMeasurementGroup.com. Six of the 27 projects share, as a central theme, the goal of providing high-quality care for individuals living with HIV/AIDS who belong to groups that are traditionally underserved because of linguistic, cultural, racial, and economic barriers that prevent their full integration into the traditional service system. These six projects formed a working group to share innovation in service delivery strategies.

This article grows out of the Community-Based Organizations (CBO) Work Group of the HRSA SPNS Cooperative Agreement. The aim of the article is to provide technical assistance to other CBOs providing or hoping to provide services to people with HIV/AIDS. The demands of providing services are complex, and they constantly change with new medical knowledge and fluctuations in the political and economic landscape. The six organizations represented in the CBO Work Group offer their experiences and lessons learned after the first three years of designing and implementing model projects to reduce barriers to care for individuals and disenfranchised groups living with HIV/AIDS. Table 1 gives a summary of the six projects.

TABLE 1. The Six Projects of the CBO Work Group

Project	Grant Title	Description
Center for Community Health, Education, and Research (CCHER)/Haitian Community AIDS Outreach Project (Dorchester, Massachusetts)	Enhanced Innovative Community and Hospital-based Case Management Program	The Center for Community Health, Education and Research/Haitian AIDS Project (CCHER/HAP) of Dorchester, Massachusetts seeks to enhance its current community and hospital-based case management system. The enhancement adds one-on-one intensive counseling sessions and educational training to its current system of care. CCHER has developed a Haitian culturally competent risk reduction curriculum. Clients come from the Haitian population residing in the Greater Boston Area who are HIV-positive or have AIDS.
The Fortune Society (New York, New York)	Discharge Planning and Case Management for Latino and Latina Prisoners Who Are HIV-Positive and Symptomatic	The Fortune Society delivers culturally and linguistically appropriate services to Hispanic women and men prisoners and releasees who are HIV-positive and symptomatic in New York City jails and New York state prisons. This project focuses on discharge planning for prisoners, case management referrals with follow-up, and intensive case management post release, including support in making the transition from prison to community. This innovative approach entails identification of and consistent contact with clients prior to release.
Larkin Street Youth Center (San Francisco, California)	HIV Service Delivery Model for Homeless Youth and Young Adults, 16 to 26 Years of Age, with CDC Defined Stage III and IV AIDS	There are two primary objectives for this project. First, the Larkin Street Youth Center (LSYC) has expanded their existing "Aftercare" program services which provide emergency housing, comprehensive primary medical care and psychosocial support services for homeless youth living with HIV to serve CDC-defined HIV symptomatic disease or AIDS diagnosed youth. Secondly, LSYC is establishing an "Assisted Care Facility"; which will consist of a twelve-unit assisted living and long-term care facility. This permanent housing program will be a focal point for providing a coordinated service delivery model that manages the medical, substance abuse, and mental health treatment needs of these young people. The cadre of services to be provided include: (1) Social Services–case management, mental health and psychiatric care, counseling, advocacy; (2) Health Services–direct provision of HIV primary healthcare, TB screening, nutrition counseling; (3) Personal Care Services–nutrition, food vouchers, clothing, transportation; and (4) Recreation and Social Activities. This facility will be open and supervised 24 hours a day.

TABLE 1 (continued)

Project	Grant Title	Description
Outreach, Inc. (Atlanta, Georgia)	A Safe Place	Outreach Inc.'s project, A Safe Place, delivers a culturally competent HIV/AIDS intervention model for addicts. Using a peer counselor and street outreach team model for service delivery, Outreach, Inc. expanded enrollment and enhanced retention of substance abusers with HIV by opening a satellite facility and drop-in center within the zip code that represented the highest incidence of HIV disease in the state of Georgia. Activities include assisting addicted HIV-infected clients in obtaining and complying with medical, substance abuse, and mental health treatments. The project also expanded services for individuals who are being discharged from correctional facilities.
PROTOTYPES (Culver City, California)	PROTOTYPES WomensLink: Reduction of Barriers to HIV/AIDS Care	PROTOTYPES heads a consortium of Los Angeles County agencies designed to be a community-based, outpatient (settlement-house) model for delivering a comprehensive continuum of services for women living with HIV/AIDS. Women are recruited throughout Los Angeles County in order to: (1) provide a range of quality services to substance abusing women with HIV designed to increase use of healthcare services and adherence to treatment; (2) change risk behaviors; (3) increase compliance with medical treatment and enhance access to existing services through outreach; (4) improve quality of life through comprehensive case management; (5) increase providers' knowledge, receptiveness and skill in treatment of women substance abusers living with HIV; (6) develop and evaluate models for replication and integration into HIV/AIDS delivery systems for women; and (7) disseminate information about successful service models.
Well-Being Institute (Detroit, Michigan)	Well-Being Institute Women's Intervention Program	The Well-Being Institute Women's Intervention Program is a comprehensive, nursing-based intervention program designed for substance abusing women with HIV who are not accessing existing health delivery systems. The program is two-tiered; tier one services assist women in overcoming access barriers to primary healthcare services; tier two services focus on becoming drug free and providing housing for the women and their children.

CBO WORK GROUP CONSENSUS ON BASIC TENETS OF COMMUNITY CARE

While the six CBO grantees differ markedly from one another in terms of their service focus, population focus, and geographical area, a key element that unites them is the reduction of barriers for traditionally underserved groups. Another key element is the development of innovative model interventions for these clients. As part of their first meetings, the six projects easily reached consensus about the basic tenets of "good community care"; these basic principles to increase access and reduce barriers to service are listed in Table 2.

PROVIDER PERCEPTIONS OF BARRIERS BEFORE AND AFTER PROGRAM

With respect to service providers' perceptions of service barriers, after projects had completed their third year, they were asked to complete a qualitative evaluation that would incorporate data on barriers to services from the perspectives of project staff, focus groups of consumers, archival data, and

TABLE 2. Basic Tenets of Community Care for Increasing Access and Reducing Barriers

- Location of services needs to be accessible

- Staff need to be representative of population to be served and well trained in all relevant issues, including cultural competence

- Services need to be language-appropriate

- Outreach to consumers/clients needs to be an integral component of the programs

- Identification of needs and barriers needs to be client-centered

- Linkages to services need to be strong and real with co-location of staff where possible

- Transportation and accompaniment services need to be provided

- Child care services need to be available

- Peer support needs to be available

- Primary needs such as food and clothing need to be provided

- Assertive case management is needed to ensure strong links to medical services

advisory committees. Table 3 shows staff ratings of the extent to which 12 factors served as barriers to clients' getting services before projects began and then again, three years later.

As can be seen in Table 3, most of the specific barriers appeared to have been reduced by the third year. Barriers that were rated as the highest before projects were implemented included: (1) lack of public funding; (2) other agencies believe clients will not comply; (3) long waiting lists; (4) clients not enrolled in public assistance; (5) other agency staff insensitive, not knowledgeable, etc.; (6) other agencies do not provide services in appropriate

TABLE 3. Providers' Perceptions of Barriers to Services Before CBO Projects Began and Three Years Later[1]

Barrier	X̄ Barriers Rating Before Demonstration Project	X̄ Barriers Rating Three Years Later	Change
Lack of public funding	6.5	4.2	− 2.3
Other agencies believe clients will not comply	5.7	3.5	− 2.2
Long waiting lists	5.6	2.2	− 3.4
Clients not enrolled in public assistance	5.5	3.2	− 2.3
Other agency staff insensitive, not knowledgeable, etc.	5.2	2.6	− 2.6
Other agencies do not provide services in appropriate environment	5.2	2.7	− 2.5
Lack of transportation	4.6	1.5	− 3.1
Other agency staff feel they lack knowledge or training	4.5	1.6	− 2.9
Other agencies cannot provide appropriate language	3.7 (Spanish, Haitian Creole, Asian/PI)	2.3	− 1.4
Lack of child care	3.3 (women focused)	1.6	− 1.7
Gatekeepers not making appropri. referrals	1.5	< 1	
Other	1.3	1	

[1]Responses ranged/rated on scale of 1-7.

environment; (7) lack of transportation; and (8) other agency staff feel they lack knowledge or training.

The barriers that were rated as most significantly reduced by the third year included: (1) lack of public funding; (2) other agencies believe clients will not comply; (3) clients not enrolled in public assistance; (4) other agencies do not provide services in appropriate environment; (5) other agency staff insensitive, not knowledgeable; (6) other agencies cannot provide appropriate language; and (7) long waiting lists. There were a number of ways the six projects worked directly and indirectly on these barriers.

With regard to "long waiting lists," most of the projects established close working relationships with other HIV-related services and assisted clients in navigating the system. In addition, a large number of new clients were able to access HIV services just by the creation of the six new CBO Work Group projects.

With regard to transportation, most of the CBO projects instituted transportation programs for their clients or collaborated with another agency that did.

With regard to agency staff not being knowledgeable or lacking training, many of the six projects provide training and technical assistance, advocacy, and participated in collaborations to impact this barrier. Line workers are the keys to daily practice reform. For example, when one of the major changes needed is to raise the priority given to substance abuse problems, the whole organization must understand and accept these changes, and senior managers can set the tone for the acceptance (or the rejection). Training for both line staff and senior managers is important. However, the CBO Work Group projects noted that the number of staff trained is far less important as an outcome measure, than what they do differently when they return to carrying out the daily practices of the organization. And training is *not* the change; after the training, consultants or technical assistance experts need to be in place to assist staff in the process of implementing change.

DATA ON CLIENTS

The six CBOs admitted 1,453 clients during the period of October 1994 to June 30, 1999. Figure 1 shows the cumulative enrollments during this period. Data regarding the sociodemographic characteristics of these clients were collected using a form developed by Huba, Melchior, staff of The Measurement Group, and the HRSA SPNS Cooperative Agreement Projects (1997a). Referred to as *Module 1: Demographics-Contact Form*, the instrument contains items pertaining to an individual's ethnic/racial background, marital, housing, and employment status, primary language, sources of income, sources of medical insurance, primary location where medical care is obtained, and recency of behaviors that put the individual and/or others at greater health risk.

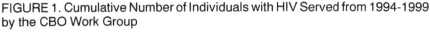

FIGURE 1. Cumulative Number of Individuals with HIV Served from 1994-1999 by the CBO Work Group

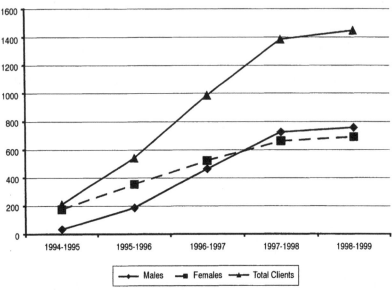

Women comprised 47.8% of the sample, men 52.2%. With regard to primary ethnicity, 67.0% of the sample was African American/Black, 21.6% Hispanic/Latino, 9.8% Caucasian, 0.8% Asian/Pacific Islander, 0.6% Native American, Aleutian, Native Alaskan, 0.2% unknown. The client's primary language was 85.7% English, 8.5% Spanish, 5.0% Haitian Creole, 0.1% French, 0.6% Other/Not Indicated.

With regard to children, the women had an average of 2.05 children (*SD* = 1.76); 49.6% of the children were living with the women at the time of enrollment, and 73.1% of them needed care while the women were getting services. The men had an average of 1.22 children (*SD* = 1.69); 5.4% of the children were living with the men at the time of enrollment, and 36.8% of them needed care while the men were getting services. Almost one-half (59.9%) of the entire sample was single (never been married) at the time of enrollment; 14.0% were married or living in a common law relationship.

Of the women, 84.6% identified themselves as being heterosexual, 3.9% as being lesbian, 4.8% as being bisexual, and 6.8% as being undecided or refusing to indicate their sexual orientation. Of the men, 68.6% identified themselves as being heterosexual, 12.7% as being gay, 5.8% as being bisexual, and 13.0% as being undecided or refusing to indicate their sexual orientation.

With regard to income, at the time of their enrollment into the CBO programs, most of the sample either had no identifiable income at all or was receiving income subsidized by the government. Specifically, 45.5% of the clients had no identifiable income, 19.5% were receiving SSI, 8.6% AFDC, 6.7% general relief, 6.9% Social Security, and 3.4% state disability. Approximately 7% were working either full- or part-time and were receiving wages or a salary, 2.2% were receiving employer benefits, 0.2% were receiving private payer insurance, and 1.5% were receiving income from other sources (including child support and private organizational assistance). For this sample, the relationship between a client's gender and whether or not he or she had some source of income was statistically significant; more men (73.0%) than women (19.3%) tended not to have any identifiable source of income, $\chi^2(1) = 380.87$, $p < .001$.

Since their participation in the HRSA programs, 7.4% ($N = 107$) of the CBO clients changed their employment status. Of the 107 clients who changed their employment status, 65.4% were women and 34.6% were men. The relationship between change in employment status and gender was significant [$\chi^2(1) = 14.48$, $p < .001$]; more women (10.4%) than men (5.0%) changed their status over time. Note that this change does not necessarily reflect a change from being employed to not being employed or vice versa, as clients could be employed full-time or part-time, unemployed but seeking work, unemployed but not wishing to seek work, or disabled at one or more points in their enrollment history.

Many of the individuals who came to the CBO projects were engaged in behaviors that put themselves at further health risk or put others with whom they came in contact at risk for HIV, other medical conditions, or potential criminal justice involvement. In Tables 4 and 5 are distributions for the men and women with respect to their recency of drug use and "risky" sexual behaviors, respectively. Individuals who indicated that they had engaged in a behavior in the previous 30 days are counted in the percentages listed for "Current." Those individuals who had engaged in a behavior at some time in their lives but not in the last 30 days are counted in the percentage listed for "Prior." Lastly, those individuals who stated that they never engaged in a behavior noted as "No." Overall, the program enrolled individuals who tend to be underserved.

There are significant relationships between a client's gender and the recency with which he or she engages in a number of substance abuse and sex behaviors. In all cases but one (having sex with an HIV-positive partner), the chi-square value for the difference between the male and female distribution- is statistically significant ($p < .001$). For example, of those with valid data, men tended to more recently abuse alcohol, use heroin, use crack cocaine, use other illicit drugs, inject drugs and to share needles than did women. In addition, more men than women had a sexually transmitted disease more recently (other than HIV) and had unprotected sex with a female partner.

TABLE 4. Substance Use/Abuse Behaviors of Male and Female Participants

	Males	Females
Alcohol Problem	n = 455	n = 425
None	9.0%	34.1%
Prior (before last 30 days)	57.4%	37.9%
Current (within last 30 days)	33.6%	28.0%
Heroin Use	n = 470	n = 428
None	57.2%	70.8%
Prior (before last 30 days)	37.4%	22.7%
Current (within last 30 days)	5.3%	6.5%
Crack Cocaine Use	n = 459	n = 425
None	21.1%	36.3%
Prior (before last 30 days)	54.2%	37.9%
Current (within last 30 days)	24.6%	25.9%
Other Illicit Drug Use	n = 471	n = 425
None	17.8%	51.1%
Prior (before last 30 days)	72.4%	38.2%
Current (within last 30 days)	9.8%	10.7%
Injects Drugs	n = 469	n = 592
None	53.1%	69.9%
Prior (before last 30 days)	42.6%	26.5%
Current (within last 30 days)	4.3%	3.5%
Shares Needles for Injection Drug Use	n = 451	n = 581
None	57.6%	75.6%
Prior (before last 30 days)	37.9%	22.5%
Current (within last 30 days)	4.4%	1.9%

However, more women than men participated in sex work more recently and had unprotected sex with a male partner.

Another interesting characteristic about the individuals who were enrolled by the projects is their involvement in the criminal justice system. As can be seen in Table 6, approximately 80 percent (87.5%) of the men had at some point in their lives been involved with the criminal justice system, while only one-half (51.2%) of the women had been. This relationship between recency of criminal justice system involvement and gender is statistically significant ($p < .001$).

IDENTIFICATION OF BARRIERS TO SERVICE ACCESS

As part of their participation in the HRSA SPNS Cooperative Agreement, the six CBO projects agreed to collect data on perceived barriers to services. These

TABLE 5. Sex Behaviors Engaged in by Male and Female Participants

	Males	Females
Sex Work/Survival Sex	n = 450	n = 564
None	78.0%	56.7%
Prior (before last 30 days)	18.4%	34.8%
Current (within last 30 days)	3.6%	8.5%
Has STD (other than HIV)	n = 451	n = 533
None	18.6%	45.0%
Prior (before last 30 days)	78.3%	49.9%
Current (within last 30 days)	3.1%	5.1%
Sex With an Injection Drug User	n = 226	n = 442
None	39.8%	53.8%
Prior (before last 30 days)	55.3%	40.5%
Current (within last 30 days)	4.9%	5.7%
Unprotected Sex With Males	n = 451	n = 594
None	70.3%	4.7%
Prior (before last 30 days)	25.7%	76.9%
Current (within last 30 days)	4.0%	18.4%
Unprotected Sex With Females	n = 460	n = 578
None	9.6%	80.6%
Prior (before last 30 days)	73.3%	17.1%
Current (within last 30 days)	17.2%	2.2%
Sex With Person Infected With HIV	n = 212	n = 478
None	17.0%	16.3%
Prior (before last 30 days)	69.8%	70.3%
Current (within last 30 days)	13.2%	13.4%

data were collected from both clients' and service providers' perspectives. Clients of the CBO projects completed an instrument called the *Module 4B: Barriers and Facilitators Form* (Huba, Melchior, Staff of The Measurement Group, and the HRSA SPNS Cooperative Agreement Projects, 1997b). This form contained 17 items pertaining to potential service barriers and 11 items pertaining to potential factors that might facilitate a client's getting services.

Figure 2 shows the percentage of males and females who thought that each one of the 17 items listed in the *Module 4B: Barriers and Facilitators Form* was a barrier to services.

As can be seen in Figure 2, the most frequently cited barriers were: (1) hard to get to services (transportation); (2) didn't know where to get services; (3) thought services didn't exist; (4) not eligible for free services; and (5) hard to make or keep appointments.

While providers rated lack of public funding, other agencies believing

TABLE 6. Criminal Justice System Involvement of Participants

	Males	Females
Criminal Justice System Involvement	$n = 550$	$n = 410$
Stated "Never" or Unknown	12.5%	48.8%
Ever	25.3%	32.9%
Current/Last 30 days	62.2%	18.3%

clients would not comply, long waiting lists, clients not enrolled in public assistance, and other agency staff being insensitive and not knowledgeable as the highest barriers, clients cited transportation, not knowing that services existed, where to get them, and difficulty making or keeping appointments as the most frequent barriers they encountered regarding services access. Waiting lists were seen by clients as barriers, but were cited somewhat less than those barriers mentioned above. It appears that clients most frequently reported barriers that are more structural–and need providers to provide enhanced outreach and client-patient education in order to assist underserved populations to access our service systems.

EARLY LESSONS LEARNED

Lesson 1: Defining, Refining and Modifying Plans

In the process of defining, refining, and modifying service plans, community-based organizations (CBO) are already thinking about future modifications. Because CBO staff know their populations, they can think through "escape routes" and alternative plans to meet evolving client needs. The best plans from local communities for complex multi-year service strategies require flexibility, revision and reassessment.

In light of the rapidly changing environment of HIV/AIDS services, each of the CBOs needed to critically examine its goals, project components, membership of prospective networks, and allocation of funds. In some cases this process of reassessment allowed for new and expanded directions while staying within the scope of the evaluation design. As one CBO Work Group member stated, "when you put your program together, it is different than what you expected." Another stated, "I've been able to use the proposed project as leverage to add other components. Now the model is even more comprehensive." The CBO members felt that it was important to note the tensions between wanting to provide services immediately and having sufficient time to develop all project components. In addition, it was noted that developing language-appropriate materials and research instruments took considerable time (see "Lesson 4: Cultural Considerations" following) and needed support from the funding agencies.

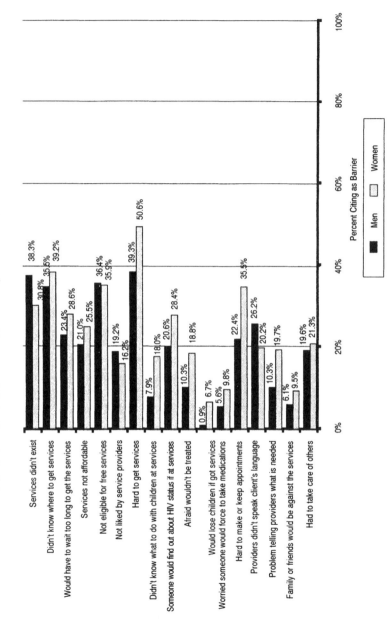

FIGURE 2. Barriers to Services Cited by Clients at Enrollment

In many communities, multiple changes are under way as part of welfare reform, community development, implementation of managed care approaches to healthcare, and medical advances. In some communities impacted by HIV/AIDS, and where multiple agency service infrastructures have been established, these initiatives are often placed in the position of competing with each other for publicity, elected officials' support, volunteers, grants, and other resources. If these parallel efforts and resources could be coordinated in some way, optimal impact could be achieved. However, coordinating all these efforts is a major task and cannot easily be done by one project within the scope of its original goals and objectives.

Lesson 2: Increasing Access, Reducing Barriers
Leads to Increased Need to Utilize Services Appropriately

The CBO Work Group projects all found that as some barriers go down, others go up. Once we increase access and a participant/client enters and is comfortable with the system, we identify more needs than had been anticipated. This can lead to increased burdens on staff time and potentially overwhelm the program. For example, just as effective outreach services succeed in increasing access to services for disenfranchised populations with more complex needs, case management services are needed to assist clients in using services appropriately, particularly primary care services.

As one CBO project director stated, "Before there was HIV/AIDS we all were here with all 'our baggage'–with all our problems and needs–including work, childcare, and/or all the things that people try to escape. Now these problems are back on the table. Our clients need to know that this is Life 101–'Welcome Back to the Norm.' Our job is to assist them in learning skills to cope with all the struggles. We need to help clients see all the options, life skills, consequences, and opportunities."

Lesson 3: Consumers as Staff

Many of the CBO Work Group projects hired recovering staff, staff living with HIV/AIDS, ex-offender/ex-sexworker staff, etc. It is important for staff to have an adequate time for stabilization. For recovering staff, CBOs often require two years "Clean and Sober." However, for staff living with HIV/AIDS often there is little time before they are taking on incredible responsibilities. Further the projects frequently experienced periods of turmoil, as staff became ill.

It was also noted that staff turnover doesn't always mean that the project is weakened. It can mean that the project can keep getting stronger. CBO Work Group members discussed need for staff support groups, cross-training, and staff rotations. A number of the CBOs rotated staff into different programs in order to give them a break from the daily stresses of direct HIV/AIDS services. The Fortune Society offers an eight-week Peer Education Training Program to consumers interested in becoming peer educators. WomensLink offered a vocational training program designed to develop a pool of trained peers for a variety of available positions.

Lesson 4: Cultural Considerations

Utilization of services tends to concentrate on those who know best how to access the system. The CBO Work Group members all had implemented components that addressed cultural considerations in the broadest sense–populations of color, immigrant populations, substance abusers, adolescents, women, etc. One of the projects is working with the immigrant Haitian population in Boston.

Educating the consumer about accessing services that are appropriate for them can cut costs. For some of the immigrant populations, clients may go from provider to provider with little benefit. Consumers need to know what services are available, which services match their needs, where these services are located, and what to expect when they get there.

Adequate time for the development of language-appropriate and age-appropriate materials and evaluation instruments must be included in the planning phase of project development. CBO Work Group members noted that the length of time for this task was often underestimated.

Lesson 5: Client Issues and Medications

As more clients and staff become involved in highly active antiretroviral therapy, the CBO Work Group identified the need to monitor the impact of these new therapeutic approaches on service delivery strategy. With newer medications, clients may experience better health outcomes, but it is important to remember that some clients will not do better under these health regimens, and that we need to provide services that are sensitive to them as well.

Highly active antiretroviral therapy requires clients to adhere to complicated medical regimens, wherein specific diet restrictions have to be maintained, as does the timing of taking the medications. The CBO Work Group projects have instituted a number of strategies to assist clients who may have difficulty taking the medications.

The issue of medications also brings up the issue of "non-compliance," particularly for populations such as substance abusers. The CBO Work Group felt strongly that providers recognize that "non-compliance" has very negative connotations. It is suggested that we consider the use of the concept of "level of engagement" rather than "non-compliance," and that we train staff/providers regarding the difficulties of "complying" with complex medical regiments.

Finally, after engaging in a program regimen, clients do not want to leave services. They may drop out for awhile, but they still consider themselves part of the program. CBO staff also do not want to "terminate" services with these clients. The CBO Work Group felt there was a need to identify another level of intervention for this issue. A related issue arose for the adolescent population. Some young clients are "aging out" (over 23 years) of the adolescent category but they may be getting more ill. In this case, the adolescent providers that have the ongoing relationship may have difficulty transferring the young adult to an "adult" provider who may be mistrusted by the young adult and where an age sensitive approach is absent.

Lesson 6: Information Sharing

The ability to meet as a group (CBO Work Group) and share ideas, problems, issues and solutions demonstrated one strength of the cooperative agreement model–peer technical assistance. The Cooperative Agreement model provides an action learning process wherein the results and problems of individual projects continue to inform and enhance the progress of other projects. Since the group is an affinity group providing peer-to-peer learning and support, it is important that funders and national evaluators understand that they do not need to always be present. In fact, sometimes their presence is a barrier.

KEY ELEMENTS IN REDUCING BARRIERS AND INCREASING ACCESS TO SERVICES

Based on evaluation data and staff input, the CBO Work Group projects believe that there are four key elements to reducing barriers and improving outcomes for persons living with HIV/AIDS; these are Environments, Connections, Integrated Services, and Leveraging Funding.

Environments. Environmental considerations noted by the CBO Work Group included location of services, safety, "community space," and therapeutic design. All six of the projects centered their services within the communities they were trying to reach. However, it is important to note that a number of the projects also provide extensive outreach services that reach well beyond a single community.

One of the projects (Larkin Street) has as its major goal to establish an Assisted Care Facility for youth with late-stage AIDS. In designing and implementing this facility for youth in downtown San Francisco, the staff of Larkin Street spent two years in capitol development, planning and construction in order to come up with a truly nurturing and therapeutic environment. The color, space, and light of the facility were all chosen with its population in mind.

PROTOTYPES WomensLink was quite successful in bringing in hundreds of women to its program. However, this also meant that they outgrew their project space and then had to move. While the move was disruptive, the new environment is larger, brighter, with more "community space"–including a separate space for the women to create their own programming without staff.

Outreach, Inc. opened its "Safe Place," a drop-in center located near three housing developments in Atlanta. Outreach, Inc., uses peers to locate substance abusers living with HIV/AIDS at community sites, including public health clinics and detention centers.

Staff of the Center for Community Health, Education, and Research (CCHER) has learned that flexibility in where and how culturally competent interventions are delivered is key to making progress with enrolled clients. The agency itself is located geographically in the heart of the Haitian community, yet it is a small, nondescript building that has no identifying markers that would indicate that it is an AIDS service organization. There is no agency sign on the outside of the building, and it could easily be mistaken for someone's home, if not for the parking lot located in the rear of the building. This is a critical "environmental element" for the Haitian community that CCHER serves. The local Haitian community is tightly knit, and if clients sense that their confidentiality in seeking HIV services may be threatened if they happen to be seen entering a building known to be an AIDS service organization, it may inhibit them from seeking services.

Connections. Connections or relationships are a key consideration in behavior change. These relationships include connecting through staff, networks and consortia, referrals, case management, and training. The six agencies share both a client-focus and a relationship focus.

For all the importance of treatment protocols, levels of care, and managed care coverage, it is sometimes possible to lose sight of the reality that treatment is about human beings. The connection between a counselor, a peer helper, an outreach worker, and a person living with HIV/AIDS is a profound bond that rests as much on human relationships as on programmatic design. That workers succeed in helping individuals and families change their lives as often as they do is remarkable. That they keep trying to make a difference in their lives is equally remarkable.

Three of the projects–The Fortune Society, Outreach, Inc., and PROTOTYPES WomensLink–have established direct links with prisons and jails. The Fortune Society has as its goal providing services to Latino/Latina prisoners living with HIV/AIDS. The staff of The Fortune Society has been able to attend parole revocation hearings in advocating alternatives to re-incarceration and in obtaining "revoke and restore" dispositions for project clients detained by order of the Board of Parole. These hearings have in the past been closed, but staff were successful in overcoming this barrier mainly by utilizing their established relationship with parole officers. Prior relevant experience with the criminal justice system has been essential for The Fortune Society's success in reducing institutional barriers to reaching special inmate groups. Outreach, Inc. has established programs with both Atlanta City Jail and Fulton County Detention Center.

The CCHER project has as its focus the Haitian Community and the staff has spent much time in establishing trust, comfort, and respect with the community. This interpersonal connection between staff and client is critical. Utilizing a psychoeducational format and case management services, the Haitian staff has been able to reduce barriers and increase access to services. Because of the trust established, CCHER staff has been able to assess the extent of substance use/abuse in the community and begin to provide services for this problem.

The Well-Being Institute has developed the concept of "Hyperlink" (Anderson, Smereck, Hockman, Ross, & Ground, 1999) to describe their move to intensify connections. Utilizing a nursing-model of care for women who are living with HIV/AIDS and are substance abusers, the staff provides transportation and links the women into primary care throughout Detroit. Well-Being Institute has long-standing relationships with providers that allow clients to avoid red tape and scheduling delays. If clients have to wait, the opportunity to get them into primary care may be lost.

Integrated services. All six projects recognized that whatever population they focused upon in their proposals, most of their clients had a number of problems in addition to HIV/AIDS, including substance abuse, mental illness, physical and sexual abuse, and homelessness. Brown (1997) has described the need for integrated services for women with "multiple vulnerabilities"; i.e., that in order to truly meet the needs of a population with multiple disorders/problems, providers need to design systems that reduce fragmentation and provide multiple levels of engagement. While the concept of integrated services is not new, there are many barriers to the implementation of this design. The challenges fall into three broad categories: structural/organizational issues related to the public systems and communities in which these service entities exist; clinical issues; and consumer issues.

Some interventions place "added burden" on clients who already have high levels of burden (Brown, Huba, & Melchior, 1995). Some of the clients seen by the CBO Work Group projects cannot easily participate in structured and rigidly scheduled programs. Sometimes a client doesn't keep a scheduled appointment because he couldn't remember when or where the appointment was to occur, or because her partner beat her up, or because she was hallucinating, or because she became frightened. It is easy to state that a client is "unable or unwilling to participate" or "non-compliant"; it is more difficult and time consuming to assess the reasons a client may not be able to withstand institutional barriers. Multi-service drop-in centers allow clients to self-select treatment modality and frequency.

Leveraging funding. Innovative models require more resources, including expanded training, addressing transportation issues, addressing treatment needs of children and family members as well as the individual living with HIV/AIDS, and increased treatment slots. All six projects have been able to bring in additional funding for their projects.

One of the concerns regarding funding that was experienced by the CBO work group was the issue of the redirection of money away from effective, needed, and sensitive psychosocial services to medication-based medical treatments. The six projects were aware that: (1) given the successes of highly active antiretroviral therapy, (2) the costs of such therapy, and (3) the finite resources and resource allocations, many of the medical providers would argue for increased resources for medical services often at the expense of psychosocial services.

Advances in medical therapies will actually necessitate an increased investment in the psychosocial services that assist disenfranchised population groups in accessing treatment. The CBO Work Group projects' collective experiences suggest that a re-direction of resources to medical treatments may result in raising the barriers that have been lowered. This would be counter productive to ensuring positive health outcomes for disenfranchised groups that need the critical support services that enable them to access, be educated about, understand, and be willing to participate in and adhere to medical care. These services must not be sacrificed.

REFERENCES

Anderson, M. B., Smereck, G. A. D., Hockman, E. M., Ross, D. J., & Ground, K. J. (1999). Nurses decrease barriers to healthcare by "hyperlinking" multiple-diagnosed women living with HIV/AIDS into care. *Journal of Nursing AIDS Care, 10* (2), 27-37.

Brown, V. B. (1997). *Untreated health problems for women diagnosed with serious mental illness.* PROTOTYPES Systems Change Center.

Brown, V. B., Huba, G. J., & Melchior, L. A. (1995). Level of Burden: Women with more than one co-occurring disorder. *Journal of Psychoactive Drugs, 27* (4), 339-346.

Huba, G. J., Brown, V. B., & Melchior, L. A. (1995). Fax-in forms as a technology for evaluating community projects: An evaluation of HIV risk reduction. *Education and Psychological Measurement, 55* (1), 75-83.

Huba, G. J., Melchior, L. A., Staff of The Measurement Group, and the HRSA SPNS Cooperative Agreement Projects (1997a). *Module 1: Demographics-Contact Form.* Available online at www.TheMeasurementGroup.com.

Huba, G. J., Melchior, L. A., Staff of The Measurement Group, and the HRSA SPNS Cooperative Agreement Projects. (1997b). *Module 4B: Barriers and Facilitators Form.* Available online at www.TheMeasurementGroup.com.

Huba, G. J., Larson, T., Marconi, K., Melchior, L. A., Brown, V., Thompson, C.,

Wolfe, L., Steinberg, J., Swift, R., Gallagher, T., Jean-Louis, E., Henderson, R., Driscoll, M., Chase, P., Falus, G., Bartlett, J., Stanton, A., Anderson, L., Thomas, L., Cruz, H., McDonald, S., Rips, J., Anderson, D., Henderson, H., German, V., Grace, C., Uldall, K., Cherin, D., Meredith, K., & Smereck, G. (1996). *27 innovative models of HIV care: A summary report of first year progress.* U.S. Department of Health & Human Services, Public Health Service, Health Resources and Services Administration.

Huba, G. J., Larson, T., Marconi, K., Melchior, L. A., Brown, V., Thompson, C., Wolfe, L., Steinberg, J., Swift, R., Gallagher, T., Jean-Louis, E., Henderson, R., Driscoll, M., Chase, P., Falus, G., Bartlett, J., Stanton, A., Anderson, L., Thomas, L., Cruz, H., McDonald, S., Rips, J., Anderson, D., Henderson, H., German, V., Grace, C., Uldall, K., Cherin, D., Meredith, K., & Smereck, G. (1997). *27 innovative models of HIV care: A summary report of second year progress.* Technical Monograph Series from The Measurement Group–PROTOTYPES Evaluation and Dissemination Center for the HRSA SPNS Innovative Models of HIV/AIDS Care.

Integrating and Utilizing Evaluation in Comprehensive HIV Care Programs

Karen Richardson-Nassif, PhD
Karen L. Meredith, RN, MPH
Trudy A. Larson, MD
Linda M. Mundy, MD
Lisa A. Melchior, PhD

SUMMARY. In healthcare programs for people with HIV/AIDS, the use of evaluation data is often considered to be non-essential to the healthcare delivery system. Three innovative healthcare programs have developed specialized evaluation models within a comprehensive continuum of care. This article describes methodologies for implementing evaluation and uses of evaluation data to improve clinic programs. Data were used to ensure quality of care and that patient needs were being met, patient management, evaluation of program priorities, resource al-

Karen Richardson-Nassif is affiliated with the Department of Family Practice, University of Vermont, Burlington, VT. Karen L. Meredith and Linda M. Mundy are affiliated with the Washington University School of Medicine, St. Louis, MO. Trudy A. Larson is affiliated with the University of Nevada School of Medicine, Reno, NV. Lisa A. Melchior is affiliated with The Measurement Group, Culver City, CA.

Address correspondence to: Karen Richardson-Nassif, PhD, University of Vermont and State Agricultural College, 235 Rowell, Burlington, VT 05405-0068.

This work was supported in part by the Health Resources and Services Administration (HRSA), HIV/AIDS Bureau (HAB), Special Projects of National Significance (SPNS) Grant No. 5 U90 HA 00026-05 (University of Vermont), 5 U90 HA 00042-05 (Washington University), 5 U90 HA 00038-05 (University of Nevada), and 5 U90 HA 00030-05 (The Measurement Group). The contents of this publication are solely the responsibility of the authors and do not necessarily represent the official view of the funding agency.

[Haworth co-indexing entry note]: "Integrating and Utilizing Evaluation in Comprehensive HIV Care Programs." Richardson-Nassif, Karen et al. Co-published simultaneously in *Drugs & Society* (The Haworth Press, Inc.) Vol. 16, No. 1/2, 2000, pp. 75-86; and: *Evaluating HIV/AIDS Treatment Programs: Innovative Methods and Findings* (ed: G. J. Huba et al.) The Haworth Press, Inc., 2000, pp. 75-86. Single or multiple copies of this article are available for a fee from The Haworth Document Delivery Service [1-800-342-9678, 9:00 a.m. - 5:00 p.m. (EST). E-mail address: getinfo@haworthpressinc.com].

location and availability of future funding. It is recommended that programs that wish to implement and utilize program evaluation in clinical settings not only track health outcomes, but obtain patient feedback, monitor program operations and request appropriate resources for this process. *[Article copies available for a fee from The Haworth Document Delivery Service: 1-800-342-9678. E-mail address: <getinfo@haworthpressinc.com> Website: <http://www.HaworthPress.com>]*

KEYWORDS. Evaluation, healthcare, HIV, utilization review

INTRODUCTION

Many medical centers are developing comprehensive care programs for people living with HIV/AIDS. However, evaluating the effectiveness of these programs often is a secondary priority and difficult to implement (Meredith, Larson, Richardson-Soons, Grace, Fraser, Mundy, Melchior, & Huba, 1998; Huba & Melchior, 1996; Melchior & Huba, 1996). Evaluation data can improve program infrastructure and quality of care. Through systematic use of evaluation, program accountability is enhanced and patient health outcomes can be documented (Owen & Rogers, 1999). Due to decreasing healthcare resources, there is greater need to identify the most critical aspects of healthcare delivery. By evaluating these programs, areas of priority emerge.

Since 1995, three projects funded as Special Projects of National Significance (SPNS) by the Health Resources and Services Administration have been providing comprehensive services for people living with HIV/AIDS and evaluating the effectiveness of their programs. The three programs are the University of Vermont and State Agricultural College's Rural HIV Service Delivery Program (Grace, Richardson-Soons, Rolley, Kutzko, Alston, & Ramundo, in press; Grace, Richardson-Nassif, Rolley, Kutzko, Alston, & Ramundo, this volume), the University of Nevada School of Medicine's Early Nutrition Intervention Program (Brunner, Larson, Huba, Melchior, & Scott, this volume) and the Washington University, St. Louis, School of Medicine's Helena Hatch Special Care Center for Women (Jeffe, Meredith, Mundy, & Fraser, 1998; Meredith & Bathon, 1997; Meredith, Jeffe, Fraser, & Mundy, this volume). Each of these programs uses a variety of techniques to assess patient needs and satisfaction, and medical outcomes. Major programmatic features of each of these programs are highlighted in Table 1. Additional information about these programs is available on the Internet at www.The MeasurementGroup.com/edc_main.htm. A description of each of the three programs follows.

Vermont. The University of Vermont program provides comprehensive healthcare to all people living with HIV/AIDS throughout rural Vermont. The

TABLE 1. Summary of Comprehensive Healthcare Project Service Models and Target Populations

	University of Vermont	University of Nevada	Washington University
Brief description of population	Community-based comprehensive healthcare using satellite clinics	Nutrition program set in community-based comprehensive HIV care clinic	One-stop comprehensive HIV care in an academic medical setting
Gender	74% male	84% male	100% female
Race	88% Caucasian	76% Caucasian	77% African American
Geographic location	Rural	Suburban	Primarily urban
Median age	40 years	39 years	29 years old
Number of clients receiving care	126	147	249
HIV risk	64% men having sex with men	64% men having sex with men	Heterosexual contact
Percentage of population with IDU risk	23%	28%	6%

Note. IDU = injection drug use

project supports three statewide rural HIV/AIDS specialty clinics housed in community hospitals. An HIV/AIDS infectious disease specialist, an MD, an HIV trained nurse practitioner, a hospital social worker and a regional AIDS Service Organization representative staff the clinics. The clinics also serve as teaching platforms for community primary care providers. This project eliminates many of the barriers people living with HIV/AIDS face in rural communities: long travel distances to receive healthcare, perceived lack of confidentiality, limited number of primary care providers with familiarity to the illness and limited local psychosocial support. This program offers state-of-the-art healthcare services at one location within rural communities. The program also provides total case management for patients by integrating medical care with clinic-based social work and support from the local AIDS Service Organizations. All patients receive comprehensive medical and psychosocial care. The majority of patients that these clinics service are living in rural areas throughout Vermont, have limited access to public transportation and specialty medical care, and are primarily unemployed (Grace, Richardson-Nassif, Rolley, Kutzko, Alston, & Ramundo, 2000).

Nevada. The University of Nevada School of Medicine's Early Nutrition Intervention in HIV and AIDS Program provides comprehensive nutrition assessment and intervention services to people living with HIV/AIDS. The program is located within a comprehensive care HIV clinic. Nutrition services are offered as part of a comprehensive clinical evaluation that includes psychosocial and financial needs assessments. An integrated team approach of physicians, nurses, social worker, pharmacist, and nutritionists work together to develop a patient care plan. In addition, a nutrition risk profile developed for each patient is used to individualize needed nutrition services. The primary patient outcomes of the project are to maximize health and immune function through optimal nutrition, prevent or slow weight loss that occurs as HIV infection progresses, help manage weight gain and metabolic side effects (diabetes, hyperlipidemias), identify and address nutritional deficits, and reduce medication side effects through nutritional intervention. The innovative feature of this model is its early identification of potential or actual nutritional risk and the establishment of a protocol that can address changing nutritional needs.

St. Louis. The Washington University School of Medicine's Helena Hatch Special Care Center (HHSCC) is an integrated system of care for women living with HIV/AIDS in metropolitan St. Louis, southern Illinois, and southeastern Missouri. The center provides integrated comprehensive HIV primary and subspecialty care for women including medical care, patient education, obstetrical and gynecological care, nutrition, individual and group counseling, and spiritual care at a single site (Smits, Goegen, Delaney, Williamson, Mundy, & Fraser, in press). The nurses play an essential role in continuous monitoring of patients' health, medication adherence, and laboratory results. They also coordinate appointments for medical procedures and provide on-going patient education. Case management services are integrated with medical care to arrange transportation and facilitate referrals to resources provided by other local programs. The unique features of this program include: (1) central location combining state-of-the-art multispecialty tertiary care with primary, community-based services; (2) coordinated, comprehensive care provided in a "one-stop-shop" format; (3) immediate access to referral from testing sites, thereby reducing time to access of treatment; (4) concomitant care of women and their HIV-infected children; and (5) the provision of technical assistance and information on women and HIV to other providers within the institution and community.

Together, the three comprehensive healthcare projects enrolled 590 patients between October 1994 and March 1999. Collectively, the patients were 37.5 percent male (note that one project treats only women) with a mean age of 33.6 years (standard deviation of 1.6 years, ranging from 15 to 75 years of age). The projects varied in ethnicity, geographic distribution, age, and HIV risk factors. In one project, more than two-thirds (77.4 percent) of the enrolled patients were people of color, whereas the other two projects, the ratio of ethnic-cultural minorities among patients was essentially the reverse.

These three programs deliver comprehensive healthcare and social services, yet differ in the formats used to provide the care. Together, all three projects implemented rigorous patient and program evaluations within unique medical settings. This paper describes the evaluation processes and key findings that these three programs used to develop, modify and measure effectiveness of comprehensive HIV care.

METHODS

These three projects were required by the federal government to implement local as well as cross-cutting evaluations of their service models. ′

Cross-Cutting Evaluation

Various evaluation methodologies were used by the three projects to assess substance abuse and other patient risk factors. As part of their participation in the cooperative agreement, the projects also participated in a cross-cutting evaluation (Huba, Melchior, Larson, & Panter, this volume; Meredith, Larson, Richardson-Soons, Grace, Fraser, Mundy, Melchior, & Huba, 1998). This evaluation process required the consistent use of core data collection tools and was designed to standardize information from all three projects. All projects collected patient information including demographics, HIV risk factor assessment, health status indicators, and service utilization. These three projects had the shared goals of improving health-related quality of life, patient satisfaction with care, and maintaining overall health status.

Local Evaluation

Each project had a local evaluation design to address the specific goals and objectives of its service model. The designs of these program evaluations were diverse to address the unique components of each project, although the projects collected similar data. Table 2 shows the various evaluation methods used by the projects, some of which are project-specific and others part of a pooled multisite evaluation strategy. Each project collected both process and outcome data. Informal evaluation methods were also included in these processes, through on-site discussions with both patients and staff. Formal quarterly meetings of project representatives from the local groups served as a source of information exchange to assess program effectiveness. Together, these methodologies helped to identify the core elements required to effectively provide comprehensive care for patients with HIV.

As a group, the comprehensive care projects decided to supplement the core cross-cutting data collection instruments (Huba & Melchior, 1995) with specialized evaluation measures. In collaboration with The Measurement Group, a key informant study was designed mid-course through the five-year period to elicit the perceptions of key stakeholders in each of the three project models. The key informant assessment was developed and implemented as a semi-structured telephone interview (Huba & Melchior, 1998). The interview was designed to obtain information about the progress of these projects in areas such as patient recruitment and retention, accessibility, quality of care, education and training, consumer involvement, development of service networks, and information dissemination. The survey evaluated programmatic knowledge, perceived importance and program success for a set of 29 program elements. This information allowed the projects to acknowledge their strengths, identify areas of improvement and define essential program elements for future planning.

CLINICAL AND ADMINISTRATIVE USES OF EVALUATION DATA

By combining data from the categories above, the comprehensive healthcare projects together with The Measurement Group have identified how

TABLE 2. Evaluation Strategies Utilized by the Three Comprehensive Healthcare Projects

	University of Vermont (Rural Issues)	University of Nevada (Nutrition Issues)	Washington University (Care for Women with HIV)
Common Evaluation Strategies	• Patient characteristics • Patient behaviors (risk factors and substance abuse) • Service utilization (medical and social)	• Medical health status • Quality of life • Patient satisfaction • Program impact (key informant survey)	• Referrals • Medications • Entry/retention
Unique Evaluation Strategies	• Travel time • Travel distance • Transportation issues • Access to local HIV MD • Confidentiality	• Nutrition evaluation (physical exam) • Nutrition risk • Patient feedback on program • Referral providers attitude/knowledge of program	• Initial needs assessment • Clinical and behavioral outcomes • OB/GYN tracking • HAART/ART use
Methods	• Interviews • Questionnaires • Phone surveys	• Interviews • Questionnaires • Focus groups	• Interviews • Questionnaires

evaluation processes can meet patient, community and administrative needs for future planning of comprehensive HIV programs. For example, the review of medical information has been used to assure that state-of-the-art care is provided to all patients and areas of needed medical and psychosocial care are identified and coordinated (Jeffe, Meredith, Mundy, & Fraser, 1998). Information gained through patient feedback has allowed programs to review infrastructure and program effectiveness (Bersoff-Matcha, Horgan, Mundy, & Stoner, 1998; Meredith, Delaney, Horgan, Fisher, & Fraser, 1997; Meredith, Jeffe, Fraser, & Mundy, this volume; Soons, Larson, Meredith, Melchior, Grace, Fraser, Mundy, & Huba, 1998). Stakeholder feedback has permitted the programs to evaluate program priorities, resource allocation, and availability of future funding (Soons, Larson, Meredith, Melchior, Grace, Fraser, Mundy, & Huba, 1998). Table 3 illustrates how evaluation data can be used to modify programs.

Each of these projects has used patient and key informant data/feedback for continuous quality improvement within the clinics. Patient medical data is also used to ensure that patients are receiving state-of-the-art HIV care, monitoring patient perception of their quality of life and overall patient management (Bersoff-Matcha, Miller, Van Der Horst, Hamrick, Gase, Powderly, & Mundy, 1999). These feedback mechanisms have also been used to assess program effectiveness, as well as site and staff development needs.

Table 4 illustrates the consensus of the comprehensive healthcare projects as to the requirements for effective evaluation in medical settings. Of utmost importance, institutional leadership for the recognition of proven infrastructure and goals is essential. In addition, it is vital for effective program evaluation to have an in-house expert who has dedicated time to facilitate the design of data collection tools and perform data cleaning and analysis, as well as the necessary computers and software to run the appropriate programs. These program elements require adequate financial resources to enable them to happen. Program evaluation must be viewed as an essential element of projects by program staff as well as at the parent institution. Approaches that are necessary for success include consideration of how patients feel about having their personal information collected, keeping questions respectful and asked in confidential settings, and ensuring that patients feel safe and comfortable when communicating private issues with their providers. There must also be collaboration and respect between data collection/analysis staff and service providers. These relationships cannot be taken for granted, but must be fostered so there is a common understanding of the value for each member of the team. Finally, there must be on-going multidisciplinary communication between all parties involved in evaluation planning, data collection and data feedback to all members of the team.

The collection and input of accurate information is not a trivial aspect of

TABLE 3. Uses of Evaluation in Clinical Settings

Purpose	Method	Sample Finding	Impact
Obtaining Patient Input	• Interview/patient questionnaire • Phone survey • Focus groups	• Patients wanted care in local community • Patients wanted personalized, care nurturing environment • Patients wanted individual nutrition assessments/no groups; patients wanted shorter visits • Importance of confidentiality	• Set up local clinics to improve access • Individualized tailored care • One on one patient visits • Stopped educational groups • Changed protocol for nutrition visits (shorter) and increased efficiency • Changed physical environment of waiting room to protect confidentiality • Provided staff training on confidentiality
Track Health Indicators	• Standardized data elements (questionnaires, chart review, professional assessment) • Database reports	• Greater prevalence of substance abuse in patient population than realized • Unmet patient needs • IDUs/non-IDUs have different co-morbidities and service utilization patterns • Increase use but not everyone appropriate on HAART • Follow-up of HIV/non-HIV care inconsistent	• Change HIV care systems to meet individual patient needs • Develop new data systems • Implement staff training • Enhance referrals • Train staff and build referral networks • Improved assessment for HAART and tailored patient education • Implement reminder systems • Staff training
Monitoring Program Operations	• Stakeholder feedback	• High level professionals and administrators value comprehensive systems	• Validation of models

Note. IDU = injecting drug use; HAART= highly active antiretroviral therapy

these programs. All data collection forms must be reviewed by Institutional Review Boards to ensure appropriateness of evaluation procedures for implementation in clinical settings. All data collection staff receive intensive training on issues of patient confidentiality, ethical issues associated with data collection, the importance of data integrity and the value of data collection. Many hours and significant financial resources have been spent on database development, and training all personnel on the importance of accurate data collection and input. It is often difficult for medical and social work staff to prioritize data collection while trying to help patients with their medical and other needs. Constant feedback to all participating staff is necessary to ensure

TABLE 4. Requirements for Effective Implementation of Evaluation in Clinic-Based Healthcare Programs

Infrastructure	• Dedicated and committed data staff
	• Evaluation expertise
	• Computer hardware and software
	• Computers
	• Patient/Staff/Institutional commitment
	• Appropriate budgeting
	• Space
Approaches	• Staff training and continuing education
	• Staff involvement and feedback
	• Client sensitive approaches
	• Collaboration between data and service providers
	• Ongoing multidisciplinary communication for evaluation planning and implementation

continued buy-in to the data collection process and to ensure the understanding of the value of data collection. Because of these needs, each project has dedicated staff for these evaluation components and these staff members are available to answer questions as they arise. Therefore, for programs to benefit from this process, the appropriate resources need to be dedicated to this aspect of the program.

There is often a debate as to whether data collection makes the program a research project or allows the program to remain a service project. All three of these projects have demonstrated that the implementation and evaluation process has allowed for the tripartite academic mission of clinical excellence, education and research to be achieved. Research questions can be answered by reviewing data with and without an intervention, whether the intervention is a new treatment modality or a new service program and then comparing patient outcomes. In addition, the data points provide valuable information on patient outcomes, the services provided, program effectiveness, and areas in need of modification.

Overall and not unexpectedly, effective communication is critical in utilizing evaluation in HIV care and critical in program and evaluation implementation. It is important to use various assessment methodologies to effectively evaluate program effectiveness. Obtaining information from patients, administrators, and providers is necessary to be responsive to constant changing demands. These programs have demonstrated that evaluation findings are important to use to improve direct patient care, community networking, and service infrastructure. Evaluation as a mechanism for programmatic improvement has permitted these institutions to be more responsive to the needs of all stakeholders in the process, including patients, staff, administrators, and funders.

There are certain challenges to implementing program evaluation in these settings. First, evaluation is often perceived as a way to make criticism, by finding out what staff are not doing, doing inaccurately, or not following guidelines that are constantly changing. Second, qualitative research often needs to be repeated to determine the generalizability of the information. Third, academically-based programs may have missions different from those of community-based programs and information learned from academic settings may not be applicable to community programs. Finally, evaluation programs are resource intensive. They require dedicated, knowledgeable staff and database management. All of these factors require financial resources to make them viable.

CONCLUSION

By using a variety of data collection strategies (interviews, questionnaires, and focus groups), evaluation processes can inform patient, community and administrative issues. These data sets can also be used for quality improvement and result in modifying programs as well as strengthening institutional support. Program evaluation should be viewed as an essential requirement of all projects, if nothing else to measure health outcomes and demonstrate value of the projects. Data collection and input are not trivial aspects of program evaluation. Dedicated staff and time are required to ensure accurate information. Therefore, the authors recommend that projects that are attempting to implement and utilize comprehensive program evaluation consider obtaining patient feedback, tracking health outcomes, monitoring program operations and requesting resources to do this in the budget.

REFERENCES

Bersoff-Matcha, S. J., Horgan, M. M., Fraser, V., Mundy, L. M., & Stoner, B. P. (1998). Sexually transmitted diseases acquisition among women infected with human immunodeficiency virus type 1. *Journal of Infectious Diseases, 178,* 1174-1177.

Bersoff-Matcha, S. J., Miller, W. C., Van Der Horst, C., Hamrick, Jr., H. J., Gase, D., Powderly, W. G., & Mundy, L. M. (1999, February). *Gender differences in Nevirapine rash.* Presented at the 6th Conference on Retroviruses and Opportunistic Infections. Abstract G76, #682.

Brunner, R. L., Larson, T. A., Huba, G. J., Melchior, L. A., & Scott, B. J. (2000).

Evaluation of status and progression of HIV disease: Use of a computerized medical module. *Drugs & Society, 16*(1/2), 237-249.

Grace, C., Richardson-Nassif, K., Rolley, L., Kutzko, D., Alston, K., & Ramundo, M. (2000). Injection drug use (IDU) related human immunodeficiency virus infection in rural Vermont: A comparison with non-IDU related infections. *Drugs & Society 16* (1/2), 223-235.

Grace, C. J., Richardson-Soons, K., Kutzko, D., Alston, W. K., & Ramundo, M. Service delivery for patients with human immunodeficiency virus in a rural state: The Vermont model. *AIDS Patient Care and STDs,* 13(1): 659-666, 1999.

Huba, G. J., & Melchior, L. A. (1995). *HRSA SPNS Cooperative Agreement Module Book: Evaluation Module Summary.*

Huba, G. J., & Melchior, L. A. (1996, August). Technical and practical design issues in cross-site HIV service evaluations. In G. Huba (Chair), *Cross-site evaluations of HIV services: Technical issues and experiences.* Presented at the annual meetings of the American Psychological Association, Toronto.

Huba, G. J., & Melchior, L. A. (1998). Key informant interview for the HRSA SPNS Comprehensive Healthcare Work Group. Available online at www.TheMeasurementGroup.com/resource/struc_int.htm.

Huba, G. J., Melchior, L. A., Panter, A. T., Brown, V. B., & Larson, T. A. (2000). A national program of AIDS care projects and their cross-cutting evaluation: The HRSA SPNS Cooperative Agreements. *Drugs & Society, 16* (1/2), 5-29.

Jeffe, D. B., Meredith, K., Mundy, L. M., & Fraser, V. J. (1998). Factors associated with HIV-infected patients' recognition and use of HIV medications. *Journal of Acquired Immune Deficiency Syndromes and Human Retrovirology, 19*, 350-360.

Larson, T. A., Scott, B. J., Brunner, R. L., & Navarro, S. (1996, July). Simple nutrition evaluation measures provide clues to early intervention in weight loss. *XI International Conference on AIDS*, Vancouver.

Larson, T. A., Scott, B. J., & Brunner, R. L. (1998, July). *Effect of protease inhibitors on the nutritional health of HIV infected adults.* XII World AIDS Conference. Geneva, Switzerland.

Larson, T. A., Scott, B. J., Brunner R. L., Melchior, L. A., Huba, G. J. (1997, September). *Client ratings of nutrition services: Priorities, barriers, and integration with total HIV healthcare.* National Meeting of the Special Projects of National Significance, Washington, DC.

Melchior, L. A., & Huba, G. J. (1996, August). Issues in implementing multisite evaluations of HIV service demonstration programs. In G. Huba (Chair), *Cross-site evaluations of HIV services: Technical issues and experiences.* Presented at the annual meetings of the American Psychological Association, Toronto.

Meredith, K., & Bathon, R. (1997). Working with HIV-infected women. In M. Winiarski (Ed.), *HIV Mental Health for the 21st Century.* New York University Press.

Meredith, K., Delaney, J., Horgan, M., Fisher, E., & Fraser, V. (1997). A survey of women with HIV about their expectations for care, *AIDS Care, 9* (5), 513-522.

Meredith, K., Jeffe, D., Fraser, V., & Mundy, L. (2000). Substance abuse and health services utilization among women in a comprehensive HIV program. *Drugs & Society 16* (1/2), 185-201.

Meredith, K., Larson, T., Richardson-Soons, K., Grace, C., Fraser, V., Mundy, L., Melchior, L. A., & Huba, G. J. (1998). Building comprehensive HIV/AIDS care services. *AIDS Patient Care and STDs, (12)* 5, 379-393.

Owen, J. M., & Rogers, P. J. (1999). *Program Evaluation: From Evaluation Findings to Utilization*, pgs. 105-131.

Scott, B. J., Larson, R. A., Brunner, R. L., Navarro, S., & Mathes, M. (1999). Evolution of nutrition screening services in a community based HIV clinic. *HIV Resource Review, 3* (6), 1-8.

Smits, A. K., Goegen, C. A., Delaney, J. A., Williamson, C., Mundy, L. M., & Fraser. V. L. (in press). Contraceptive use and pregnancy decision making among women with HIV. *AIDS Patient Care and STDs.*

Soons, K. R., Larson, T. A., Meredith, K., Melchior, L. A., Grace, C. J., Fraser, V., Mundy, L. M. & Huba, G. J. (1998, November). *Using evaluation results to improve three university-based comprehensive care medical programs for HIV.* Presented at the annual meeting of the American Evaluation Association, Chicago.

A Continuum of Care Model
for Adolescents Living with HIV:
Larkin Street Youth Center

Michael Kennedy, MS, MFCC
Ronald Spingarn, MS
Anne Stanton, MSW, CSW
Mary Jane Rotheram-Borus, PhD

SUMMARY. Overcoming barriers to delivering care to adolescents living with HIV, Larkin Street Youth Center (LSYC) has developed a comprehensive HIV service delivery program. This model coordinates services for adolescents living with HIV and includes five types of services: outreach, drop-in services, routine health and medical care, dependent care, and residential/caretaking services. Stable housing was made available to youth in two settings: (1) scattered site apartments and single rooms in hotels within a small geographic area; and (2) a res-

Michael Kennedy and Anne Stanton are affiliated with the Larkin Street Youth Center, San Francisco, CA. Ronald Spingarn and Mary Jane Rotheram-Borus are affiliated with University of California, Los Angeles, CA.

Address correspondence to: Mary Jane Rotheram-Borus, Center for Community Health, UCLA, 10920 Wilshire Boulevard, Suite 350, Los Angeles, CA 90024.

This study benefited from the assistance of research staff at the Center for Community Health, Neuropsychiatric Institute, University of California, Los Angeles, including Ella Kelly, PhD; Mark Kuklinski; and Edward Hardy.

This work was supported in part by the Health Resources and Services Administration (HRSA), HIV/AIDS Bureau (HAB), Special Projects of National Significance (SPNS) Grant No. BRU900114-05 and the National Institute on Drug Abuse Grant No. 5R01DA790304. This publication's contents are solely the responsibility of authors and do not necessarily represent the official view of the funding agencies.

[Haworth co-indexing entry note]: "A Continuum of Care Model for Adolescents Living with HIV: Larkin Street Youth Center." Kennedy, Michael et al. Co-published simultaneously in *Drugs & Society* (The Haworth Press, Inc.) Vol. 16, No. 1/2, 2000, pp. 87-105; and: *Evaluating HIV/AIDS Treatment Programs: Innovative Methods and Findings* (ed: G. J. Huba et al.) The Haworth Press, Inc., 2000, pp. 87-105. Single or multiple copies of this article are available for a fee from The Haworth Document Delivery Service [1-800-342-9678, 9:00 a.m. - 5:00 p.m. (EST). E-mail address: getinfo@haworthpressinc.com].

idential care facility for disabled adolescents living with HIV. Case reports and summaries of assessments conducted with seven adolescents living with HIV are described. Clinical descriptions, health indices, and improvements in daily routines demonstrate the program's benefits; continued substance use and sexual risk acts demonstrate the need for prolonged assistance for adolescents living with HIV with comorbid disorders. *[Article copies available for a fee from The Haworth Document Delivery Service: 1-800-342-9678. E-mail address: <getinfo@haworthpressinc.com> Website: <http://www.HaworthPress.com>]*

KEYWORDS. HIV/AIDS, adolescents, continuum of care, housing

INTRODUCTION

Significant and increasing numbers of adolescents are living with HIV and are being identified at younger ages (Centers for Disease Control and Prevention [CDC], 1998a; D'Angelo, 1991; D'Angelo, Getson, Luban, & Gayle, 1991; Karon, Rosenberg, McQuillan, Khare, Gwinn, & Peterson, 1996; St. Louis, Conway, Hayman, Miller, Petersen, & Dondero, 1991). Approximately half of all new United States HIV infections are among persons younger than 25 (CDC, 1998b). Worldwide, approximately half of all cumulative HIV infections have occurred in 15- to 24 year-olds (UNAIDS, 1998). HIV treatment advances are increasing the life expectancies for infants and children living with HIV and a growing number of these children are reaching adolescence (CDC, 1998a; D'Angelo, 1991; D'Angelo et al., 1991; Karon et al., 1996; St. Louis et al., 1991). Homeless or runaway youth (Shalwitz, Goulart, Dunnigan, & Flannery, 1990; Stricof, Novick, & Kennedy, 1990; Stricof, Kennedy, Nattell, Weisfuse, & Novick, 1991), young gay males (CDC, 1998b), young females (CDC, 1998b), and minority adolescents (Bowler, Sheon, D'Angelo, & Vermund, 1992; CDC, 1998c; Gayle & D'Angelo, 1991), particularly African American females (CDC, 1998c), experience disproportionately high rates of HIV and/or AIDS cases.

High HIV infection rates among adolescents have long-term costs to society. These costs are higher relative to the costs associated with older people who become infected (Hein, 1989). Young people have higher rates of partner mixing and a longer life span. Average survival time after infection with HIV has increased (Lange, 1995; Nelson, 1996) in large part due to new treatments. As a result, the number of persons infected by each HIV-infected youth may increase, and the percentage of infected persons in his or her cohort will rise with age (Morris, Zavisca, & Dean, 1995).

As the benefits of early detection continue to mount (Rotheram-Borus,

Murphy, Coleman, Kennedy, Reid, Cline et al., 1997), interventions for adolescents living with HIV are increasingly important. If these youth adhere to medical interventions, the cost of medical care is likely to be minimized and life expectancy lengthened. Successful secondary prevention efforts will reduce the spread of the virus by these youth as well as the cost to society. Therefore, resources must be put into developing and sustaining effective systems and continuum-of-care models for delivering comprehensive services to adolescents living with HIV.

The goal of this paper is to describe the multiple levels of needs among adolescents living with HIV and a model system-of-care that utilizes a rank-ordered set of needs for these youth. The impact of the care model on seven seropositive youth is documented using case reports and the results of assessments conducted over four time points. This model is designed to assist persons who plan, provide, and evaluate services for meeting multiple levels of needs of adolescents living with HIV and to improve the effectiveness and quality of systems of care that serve these youth.

Barriers to Services for Adolescents Living with HIV

It is important that providers who serve adolescents living with HIV understand the needs of this growing population, as youth's needs are distinctly different from those of HIV-infected adults. Compared with adults, adolescents have different developmental capacities (Izard, Kagan, & Zajonc, 1984; Matlin, 1983). These capacities influence youth's concept formation, problem solving, memory, decision making, language abilities, emotional states, and abilities to understand information and to adapt effectively to social and environmental demands (Izard et al., 1984; Matlin, 1983). In part, youth's capacities are limited due to the maturation of (Izard et al., 1984) or variations in new cognitive functions (Yurgelun-Todd, 1998). In addition to cognitive development, the physiologic development of adolescent females' genitalia may increase young females' risk for sexually transmitted infections, including HIV (Hein, 1989; Moss, Clemetson, D'Costa, Plummer, Ndinya-Achola Reilly et al., 1991). Concurrent with the physical pubertal-related changes, adolescence is the developmental period where personal identity is explored, and commitments are made regarding sex, gender roles, occupational choices, and political beliefs (Archer, 1989). These choices shape the trajectory of an adolescent's future; therefore, youth's serostatus and the developmental challenges faced by HIV-infected adolescents are likely to shape the search for personal identity.

While having fewer intrapersonal resources, adolescents living with HIV must meet barriers not faced by HIV-infected adults in their receipt of medical, psychosocial, housing, and other services. Adolescents living with HIV are often excluded from or are tangential recipients of HIV service programs.

For example, only eight of 30 pediatric HIV demonstration programs funded by the Maternal and Child Health Bureau focused their services specifically on adolescents (Conviser, 1993). National, state, and local laws or ordinances, and policies at community-based agencies may hinder adolescents living with HIV from receiving care. Only four states have passed specific statutes that allow persons younger than 18 to consent to treatment for HIV infection (Parham v. J.R., 99 S.Ct.2493 (1979), and Belloti v. Baird, 99 S.Ct.3035 (1979) cited in English, 1995).

Laws or ordinances that restrict or discourage adolescents from receiving medical services are likely to result in youth receiving little or no information regarding disease prevention or treatment. Adolescents' legal status also often limits their access to a variety of other services, as documented by English (1995). First, there are very few adolescent-focused drug treatment programs, and adult drug treatment programs often do not permit enrollment of minors; without drug treatment, heroin-addicted youth are more likely to engage in survival sex and criminal acts (e.g., stealing) to support their habit. Excluding adolescents from housing programs may lead to their becoming homeless (Children's Defense Fund, 1988; U.S. Conference of Mayors, 1987) and may be associated with youth bartering sex in exchange for a place to sleep. Growing numbers of adolescents, including those who are HIV-infected, encounter substantial difficulties in locating free sources of healthcare and in obtaining private or public insurance coverage. Access to antiretroviral therapies is blocked without access to medical care. Mental health services for adolescents are extremely limited and such resources that are appropriate for adolescents living with HIV are even more scarce. Most anti-discrimination laws that protect persons with HIV, such as the Americans with Disabilities Act (1990), have focused on insurance issues or the workplace. However, adolescents living with HIV often face discrimination at schools, and more commonly, within the juvenile justice and/or foster care systems. In these situations, courts have applied different, and, in some cases, less stringent standards to protect the constitutional rights of minors than for adults. Discrimination likely creates stressful conditions for adolescents living with HIV, and stress has been shown to be an important factor in the health of HIV-infected persons (Glaser & Kiecolt-Glaser, 1987; Kemeny, 1994; Schlebusch & Cassidy, 1995). Thus, there is a range of unique barriers for access to care for adolescents living with HIV.

A Continuum of Care Model for Adolescents Living with HIV

Planning, providing, and evaluating effective services for adolescents living with HIV must be based upon a broad evaluation of youth's needs (Huba & Melchior, 1998). We suggest that adolescent providers address a rank-ordered set of needs for adolescents living with HIV (Maslow, 1987): survival, safety and security, belongingness and love, confidence and self-esteem, and self-actualization. Interventions for adolescents living with HIV must focus on establishing healthy daily routines; however, stable routines require that basic survival needs are met first and that youth perceive their daily goals in the broader context of their life goals. Adolescents living with HIV whose basic needs are not met have to spend their time finding food and shelter and are not free to attend an intervention group meeting to reduce transmission behaviors (Rotheram-Borus, Murphy, Fernandez, & Srinivasan, 1998; Schneir, Kipke, Melchior, & Huba, 1998). Housing and stable sources of support for HIV-infected adolescents are most often a prerequisite to reducing sexual risk acts (Rotheram-Borus, Feldman, Rosario, & Dunne, 1994). Delivery of HIV prevention and treatment is difficult due to adolescent life stressors, living situations, and adjustment problems. In particular, high-risk youth are often estranged from their families; therefore, involving families in these programs is not often helpful (Bettencourt, Hodgins, Huba, & Pickett, 1998). Concern over disclosing one's HIV status, dealing with stigma, inadequate coping skills for reducing substance use, and failure to practice safer sex behaviors are major barriers to staying healthy for HIV-infected youth (Rotheram-Borus et al., 1998). To address a continuum of needs, Larkin Street Youth Center developed a comprehensive and coordinated continuum of care model for adolescents living with HIV.

Larkin Street Youth Center (LSYC) is a program that attempts to address the multiple levels of needs among youth aged 12-23 years who are homeless, including adolescents living with HIV. A San Francisco, community-based non-profit agency, LSYC was founded in 1984 to divert young people from prostitution, drug dealing, and other illegal and/or potentially harmful street-survival activities. Its current mission is to "create a continuum of services that inspires youth to move beyond the streets by nurturing potential, promoting dignity, and supporting bold steps by all persons" (LSYC, 1998a).

In fiscal year 1997-1998, LSYC served approximately 2,000 homeless and runaway youth on-site including 90 adolescents living with HIV (LSYC, 1998a). Overall, 75% of the youth served by LSYC report histories of sexual or physical abuse, 67% report being unable to return home due to parents who are unwilling or unable to care for them, and 53% report histories of suicidal ideation or attempts (LSYC, 1998a).

Among the youth living with HIV served by LSYC: 5% were aged 13-17, 90% were aged 18-24, and 5% were aged 25. Most were male (81%), and 8% were transgender; 88% were gay or bisexual. Sixty percent were Caucasian, 15% Latino, 9% Black, 3% Asian Pacific Islander, and 13% multi-racial (LSYC, 1998b). Three primary subgroups were served: (1) injection drug users, (2) African American or Latino or multi-racial youth, and (3) homeless or marginally housed gay/bisexual males. These youth lived in poverty: most received no income, 80% received less than $600 per month, and none received over $900 per month; 89% were unemployed. Among the youth, clinicians at LSYC determined that 77% were dually diagnosed with HIV and substance abuse or mental illness, and 65% were diagnosed with all three conditions (LSYC, 1998b), based on DSM criteria (American Psychiatric Association, 1998).

HIV Service Model

LSYC's continuum of care model provides a comprehensive range of programs designed to help disenfranchised youth obtain the necessary skills and knowledge to take control of their lives and find lasting alternatives to street life. These programs were established to link adolescents with certain needs to a specific type of service, as summarized in Figure 1. The needs range from basic survival to self-actualization and are described on a prioritized basis:

Level 1–*Survival needs* (physiological) include food, sleep, clothes, medical treatment for acute pain, stable housing, and crisis or suicide counseling,

FIGURE 1. A Continuum of Care Model for Adolescents Living with HIV

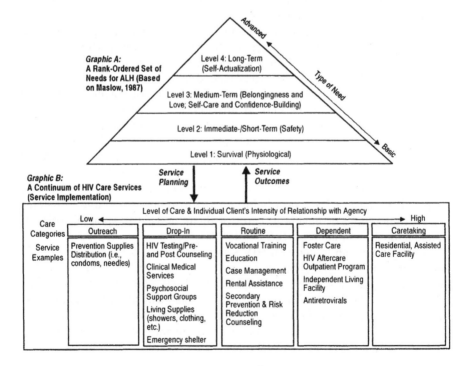

many of which are met by emergency or acute care and crisis programs. Street and community outreach are preferred service delivery methods for youth lacking immediate survival needs.

Level 2–*Immediate/Short-term needs* include protection from physical/sexual and emotional abuse, developing trust of others, protection by family/foster care/guardians, basic financial resources, one-on-one peer support, and periodic counseling. Many of these needs are met by foster care, support groups, and peer support programs. At this level, drop-in and hotline services are preferred service delivery methods for youth.

Level 3–*Medium-term needs* include self-care, confidence building, social acceptance, friendship and support networks, assertiveness, coping and interpersonal skills, peer education activities, and treatment for substance abuse and mental health. Interpersonal or interactive workshops, recreation activities, peer education programs, outpatient services, and medical care meet these needs. Antiretroviral medications for adolescents living with HIV require stabilization of youth's living situation and a strong agency/youth connection. Youth in either assisted care or residential treatment have such a relationship and, therefore, youth can start antiretroviral therapies.

Level 4–*Long-term needs,* sometimes referred to as "quality of life needs," address youth's self-sufficiency and independence. These needs may include accepting one's HIV-infection and making personal and career plans, such as starting a family, having longer-term relationships, or avoiding potentially risky situations. These needs are often met through schools, secondary prevention, career counseling/job training, family planning, and longer-term counseling programs.

Seropositive youth, particularly those who are homeless, cannot meet these basic needs for survival without a source of stable housing. Stable housing provides the bedrock for beginning to meet the higher level needs in Maslow's hierarchy. Therefore, with support from the Health Resources and Services Administration, LSYC received funding to enhance its housing program for adolescents living with HIV by adding a residential care facility for the chronically ill, which serves youth disabled by HIV or AIDS. These youth are typically comorbid for substance abuse, as well as mental health disorders, and do not have family support services as a resource. A housing assistance program was designed with two levels of care: (1) scattered site housing in individual apartments and hotel rooms in the Tenderloin District of San Francisco; and (2) a residential care facility that houses up to 12 youth and provides 24-hour healthcare, recreational and social services, vocational training, and meals. Youth in the housing assistance program receive assistance from the other LSYC programs; all are youth who are seropositive for HIV.

Restricted to seropositive youth with disabling HIV or AIDS, the residential care program is staffed by a resident manager, five counselors, a nurse/

case manager, a nutritionist, and a receptionist. On a daily basis, two to three staff members are available. All youth in the program have access to and help in adhering to antiretroviral medications, as well as the range of services described in this article. Establishing secure housing is the key to working with adolescents living with HIV and prior to establishing the residential program, there was a missing link in the assisted housing component. There was no setting in which disabled youth could obtain care.

LSYC program impact and outcome. In order to demonstrate the impact of the LSYC continuum of care model on program clients, two strategies were employed. First, the clinical team collaborated on drafting case summaries for each youth, focusing on the level of daily impairment, functioning, and quality of life. Second, assessments were conducted in individual interviews with a staff member from a university-based research organization interviewing the youth. In the first year of the program, seven disabled youth were identified and evaluated. The seven youth received housing services for one year and were available over four assessments at three-month intervals and are included in this paper. At each evaluation, the sexual and substance-use risk acts and health status, as reflected in viral loads, were obtained. The sexual behavior indices included assessments of the number of sexual partners with whom the youth engaged in vaginal and anal intercourse, and the proportion of sexual partners with whom they always had condom-protected sex acts. Assessments of substance use included specific probes using street names for the use and frequency of use of cigarettes, alcohol, marijuana, crack, cocaine, heroin, barbiturates, inhalants, and amphetamines. For each drug, the rate of use/non-use during the previous three months and the frequency of use per substance were obtained. Frequency of injecting drug use was also documented. The results of these assessments are summarized on Table 1.

Case study #1. Cyrus was removed from his biological parents' home in early adolescence because of severe physical abuse. He was placed in foster care, where he reported that he was sexually abused. He ran away from this foster placement, eventually was placed in a stable foster home, and, later, was adopted. Cyrus reports that his emotional problems were associated with truancy from school, increasing substance abuse, and acting-out behavior with his adoptive family. At the age of 17, he began to live on the streets in San Francisco, and soon thereafter, began using methamphetamines intravenously and engaging in survival sex. During this time, he came in contact with Larkin Street's Outreach team, which informed him about the agency's services.

At 17 years of age, Cyrus began to use the agency's Drop In Case Management and Medical Care programs. At age 18 he tested positive for HIV at LSYC's clinic and was referred to its Housing Assistance Program. He began

TABLE 1. Summary of Recent Sexual and Substance Use Behaviors Across Four Time Points (N = 7)

	Time 1	Time 2	Time 3	Time 4
Sexual Behaviors				
Vaginal sex				
abstinent	50.0%	71.4%	83.3%	60.0%
# of partners	1.0	2.0	1.0	2.5
> 1 partner	0.0%	50.0%	0.0%	100.0%
youth with 100% condom use	33.0%	50.0%	0.0%	50.0%
Anal sex				
abstinent	66.7%	40.0%	25.0%	50.0%
# of partners	1.5	2.0	1.3	1.0
> 1 partner	50.0%	100.0%	66.7%	100.0%
youth with 100% condom use	50.0%	67.0%	67.0%	0.0%
Substance Use				
Abstained	0.0%	0.0%	0.0%	0.0%
Youth Who Used Drugs				
Alcohol	83.0%	85.7%	85.7%	57.1%
Marijuana	57.0%	71.4%	83.3%	71.4%
Amphetamines	67.0%	57.1%	66.7%	14.3%
Heroin	25.0%	14.3%	14.3%	14.3%
Cocaine	40.0%	28.6%	33.3%	28.6%
Crack	33.0%	42.9%	50.0%	57.1%
Mean # of Times Used Drugs Among Users				
Alcohol	62.2	21.7	17.7	14.5
Marijuana	26.3	82.4	115.8	73.2
Amphetamines	6.5	23.5	22.3	10.0
Heroin	90.0	180.0	90.0	90.0
Cocaine	24.0	56.0	53.0	90.0
Crack	24.0	70.7	43.7	70.5

to receive counseling and housing services through the agency. Cyrus's emotional and substance-abuse problems were addressed through case management and referral to psychiatric services. He eventually decided to enter a drug treatment program, where he remained for one year. His viral load at the beginning of the drug treatment process was rather high (492,000), and his CD4 count was 299.

After a year of working to maintain sobriety in drug treatment programs, Cyrus moved into the residential care treatment program. Although his goals were to progress towards independence and maintain a clean and sober lifestyle, he relapsed into drug use. Because of substance use, Cyrus was asked to leave the residential care program, which he did. While sobriety is not a program requirement, obvious daily substance use that inhibits functioning, or dealing to other youth in the program are grounds for removal from the program. He later returned to the housing assistance program, which helped him obtain an apartment. With support from case management and psychiatric services, he stopped using drugs and began working toward his goals of full-time employment and education. By December 1997, he was taking antiretroviral medications and had a viral load of 4,850 and a CD4 count of 230. Because LSYC's services focus on harm reduction, Cyrus was eventually able to decrease his drug use and improve his quality of life. Over time, he was able to achieve full recovery.

Case study #2. Medina is a 19-year-old Latina, the daughter of immigrant parents. Medina reported that sexual abuse by her stepfather led her to leave stable housing at 17 and turn to the streets. Primarily dependent on alcohol, Medina traded sex for drugs and money, and was involved in violent relationships. She occasionally dropped into street outreach services at LSYC. Over time, a closer and more stable relationship was established with the agency. She tested seropositive for HIV in 1997 and entered treatment for alcohol dependence. If she had not had a place for residential stability, Medina would have returned to bartering sex and using alcohol. After treatment, she entered the residential care program and initiated antiretroviral medication. She was stabilized in residential treatment, currently her viral load is undetectable, and she has not bartered sex during the last year. She began treatment with a psychiatrist and worked through issues related to depression. She then was able to focus on taking advantage of educational and vocational services provided by the Center. Medina eventually transitioned into an independent living situation.

Case study #3. Jack was raised by a single parent who often left him unsupervised from an early age. Jack began using marijuana and alcohol before he was 13. He also skipped school and ran away from home. At age 17, he lived on the streets in San Francisco and soon started to inject methamphetamines and participate in survival sex. He was introduced to LSYC through its outreach team, and began to use its case management services. Jack tested positive for HIV at age 18, and was referred to LSYC's program for seropositive youth. He was housed through the agency's program for 2 years, during which time he made an unsuccessful attempt to stop using illicit drugs.

Before moving into the residential care facility, Jack began to reduce the amount of his substance use and to meet and work more successfully with his case manager. Jack expressed an interest in moving into the residential care facility, which motivated him to complete more of his treatment goals, including accessing medical care and beginning an educational training program. At admission in December 1997, his viral load was 11,000, and his CD4 count was 324. Jack has lived in residential care for 8 months; he has maintained stable housing, complied with house rules, further reduced his substance use, and is taking computer classes and participating in LSYC's vocational program. Jack's current viral load is 243,000, which is dangerously high, and his CD4 count is 258. Case managers are encouraging Jack to begin medication to treat his HIV infection.

Case study #4. Joshua, aged 16, was referred to the LSYC program for seropositive youth from San Francisco General Hospital's Psychiatric Ward, where he had been in the inpatient psychiatric program for two weeks and was receiving antipsychotic medications. At that time, he had already been diagnosed with AIDS. He had Kaposi's sarcoma lesions over most of his body, causing inflammation around his eyes that severely restricted his vision. Joshua was unable to speak and could only grunt. He was an active injection drug user, as well as a crack user.

Joshua was immediately housed through LSYC's program. Maintaining his housing required daily home visits by program staff, including assistance with compliance to his psychiatric medication regimen and interventions to reduce substance use. No drunken or overdose behavior was acceptable in order to remain in the program. During the nine months following his entry to the program, he refused medical care and was often unable to manage activities of daily living. As soon as LSYC's residential care facility was completed, Joshua entered the program. At admission in December 1997, his CD4 count was 8, and his viral load was 292,000. The residential program ensured that Joshua adhered to his regimen of psychiatric medications. This allowed case management staff to encourage him to begin medical treatment for AIDS, including medications and chemotherapy. Joshua has responded well to the structured, supportive housing model at LSYC's residential care program. Joshua now speaks, participates in group activities and remedial education programs, and is able to interact with staff and residents. Although Joshua continues, at times, to use drugs, the amount and frequency of his use has dramatically decreased. He continues to require assistance with activities of daily living. Joshua's current viral load is 476 and his CD4 count is 263.

While in residential care, Joshua shared some of his history with his case manager. He reported a history of physical and sexual abuse by his mother and stepfather, as well as a long history of mental illness, foster and group home placements, and a family history of mental illness. He disclosed that he began to barter sex at age 12 years, and continued to do so until entering the residential care program. Through case management and psychiatric consultation, Joshua continues to heal from his past experiences and build stronger bonds with staff and other residents.

Case study #5. Mike was born to a substance-abusing, single parent. He, his sister, and his mother were homeless throughout his childhood, leading to severe physical neglect and abuse by his mother and her boyfriend. Mike and his sister were prostituted during their childhood by his mother's boyfriend. His mother consented to this in order to obtain money for drugs. By age 15, Mike was abandoned by his mother in San Francisco, where he continued to prostitute and started injecting methamphetamine. At this point he began to use LSYC's Drop In Center and Case Management services.

At age 18, Mike tested positive for HIV and was referred to the program for seropositive youth. He received housing support and case management services. At age 19, Mike suffered his first schizophrenic episode, which led to his disconnection from LSYC services, except for his case manager's attempts to track him down. At that time, he was using crack heavily, his hygiene deteriorated dramatically, and he was so severely delusional that he could not communicate coherently. His viral load in the summer of 1997 was 308,100. Mike was eventually hospitalized for a psychotic break. He was referred back to the program for seropositive youth from the hospital after being stabilized on psychiatric medications. He was housed in a hotel, with daily home visits to assist with medication compliance and activities of daily living.

When the residential care facility opened, Mike moved in; his medication adherence improved and he began to access medical care consistently. At admission, his CD4 count was 8 and his viral load was 152,000; his viral load is now less than 50 and his CD4 count is 81. He dramatically reduced the quantity and frequency of his substance use. Mike had never learned to read; through the program's remedial education program, he is beginning to read and write simple words.

Case study #6. Stu was born to an alcoholic mother who suffered from severe depression. The mother attempted suicide by deliberately crashing her car. Stu, who also was in the car, sustained severe head trauma. He also suffered severe physical abuse and neglect and was permanently removed from his home by age 7. He was placed in a series of group homes, and by age 9 was placed in an adoptive home, where he reports that he was sexually and emotionally abused. Eventually, he was placed in a residential psychiatric facility because of severe emotional and behavioral problems. After several inpatient admissions, the abuse was disclosed and he was removed from the adoptive family, but placed with a relative of the adoptive father in the Bay Area at age 17.

Stu came to San Francisco to engage in prostitution and injecting methamphetamine use. After learning that Stu was sharing needles and engaging in unsafe sex, his foster parent contacted LSYC to request that Stu be given an HIV antibody test. With Stu's consent, Stu was tested for HIV and found to be seropositive; he was enrolled in the program for seropositive youth, received case management and housing support, and began to be treated by a psychiatrist, who supervised psychiatric and neurological testing of Stu to determine the cause of his developmental delay. Unfortunately, these tests were inconclusive, leading to difficulties in finding a suitable group home placement.

Stu moved into LSYC's residential care facility when it opened in 1997. At admission, his viral load was 2,184, and his CD4 count was 168. Since his living situation has stabilized, he has been able to comply more effectively with medications for his psychiatric issues and his HIV, has reduced his substance use, and has been able to participate in group activities and educational programs. He responds well to behavior management goals set and reinforced by residential care staff members. His current viral load is less than 50, and his CD4 count is 303.

Case study #7. Susie is the daughter of a Latina alcoholic mother. She was sexually abused as a child by her stepfather for seven years; she disclosed the abuse at age 14 but her stepfather was not imprisoned. She was also neglected as a child, and began to drink alcohol at age 9. At age 14 she ran away from home and came to San Francisco, where she used drugs and increased her alcohol use. She had several abusive relationships and bore a child at the age of 17. She lived in a single room in a San Francisco Tenderloin district hotel with her child. Upon being tested for HIV, she found she was positive. Some time later, she had another child.

At LSYC's program for seropositive youth, Susie received case management services and occasional housing assistance. Throughout 1997, Susie continued to use substances, especially alcohol. She was seen for medical care at Larkin Street's clinic and entered a drug treatment program, through which she successfully stopped using methamphetamine and other drugs, but continued to drink alcohol. When Susie was in a hospital for an operation, her boyfriend physically abused her children, and they were removed from her custody. After the removal of her children, she continued to drink heavily for several months, then reentered drug treatment.

Susie moved to the residential care facility with the goal of completing an 18-month drug treatment program, stabilizing her housing and health status, clarifying her educational goals, and regaining custody of her children. Her CD4 count at admission was 401, with a viral load of 30,000. Residing at residential care, she has accessed supportive counseling and case management services, helping her progress toward these goals. As she ages out of the program and prepares to move into a transitional housing program for single mothers in recovery, she has had a year of sobriety and has made progress in regaining custody of her children. She also has a plan for the next 2 years that includes work and education. Her current CD4 count is 646, with a viral load of 98.

Summary of case studies. Community-based agencies such as Larkin Street Youth Center strive to provide effective, high quality services that meet each of the levels of needs for adolescents living with HIV. These case studies demonstrate that each youth has a unique pattern of needs and their own pathway for achieving personal stability and productivity. These pathways affect the intensity and range of services required to meet the needs of these youth, and have important implications for systems of care that attempt to serve adolescents living with HIV.

Almost all of these youth represent failures of parenting and social service agencies. These youth have experienced severe and repetitive negative stressors, particularly abuse, neglect, and abandonment. Not unexpectedly, these youth demonstrate histories of significant impairment in daily life functioning, mental health disorders, and early substance use. Youth's lives have spiraled to the level where daily survival is questionable, and there is no safety net to provide stability. In this context, residential treatment becomes a cornerstone to providing survival needs and stability without the youth resorting to selling sex or drugs. Only in the context of stable fulfillment of survival needs can youth receive consistent support and begin to cope effectively with the significant early stressors. Because youth are likely to experience many illnesses and have no family safety nets, residential treatment is likely to be needed for a prolonged period, and change in substance use patterns and mental health problems is likely to be slow.

Transmission behaviors. Table 1 summarizes the sexual and substance-use risk acts of the adolescents living with HIV in the residential care program over four assessment periods. The sample size is too small to conduct any statistical analysis. Most youth were sexually active over time, typically with one female partner and two males in the previous three months. Most youth had engaged in unprotected sexual acts over the previous three months, and this was a pattern repeated over all assessments. All youth also engaged in substance use across time. Alcohol and marijuana were the substances most commonly used. While inspection of the mean frequency of use suggests declines in alcohol use, over time the opposite occurred for other drugs: marijuana use increased over time. Unfortunately, a facility for distribution of medical marijuana opened in the same neighborhood soon after the residential care center opened that may explain the increase. Amphetamine, crack, and cocaine use remained common, and use was frequent. One youth used heroin consistently across each assessment. These data indicate a substantial need for continued interventions for secondary prevention of HIV with adolescents living with HIV.

Substantial clinical improvement occurred for the seven clients studied in the residential care facility. Concurring with these reports are the indices of viral load obtained from medical charts. In contrast to reports of other samples of adolescents living with HIV that find only about half of the youth on antiretroviral medications (Gwadz, De Vogli, Rotheram-Borus, Diaz, Cisek, James et al., in press), all of these youth at LSYC were receiving antiretroviral medication. There were substantial improvements in physical health status as reflected in these viral indices. As new prophylactic interventions become available, adolescents living with HIV will require access to healthcare and a complementary set of personal motivations, attitudes, values, skills, and opportunities to utilize health resources. Behaviors such as adhering to medication regimens, keeping appointments with care providers, and participating in medical care decisions contribute to long-term survival of persons, including those living with HIV (Horwitz & Horwitz, 1993; O'Brien, Petrie, & Raeburn, 1992; San Francisco AIDS Foundation, 1998). The youth at LSYC are able to access these services because they are in a residential program where medical care and other needed services are immediately available.

However, the assessments of sexual and substance use indicate substantial need for reductions in these ongoing risk behaviors that place both others at risk for infection and the already infected youth at risk of reinfection. Specifically, comprehensive substance-use treatment programs are needed for these youth on a daily and ongoing basis. Many agencies are able to provide only one or two services, or at most, a patchwork of services that may not be appropriate to attract and/or retain adolescents living with HIV. Community-based agencies will not succeed in recruiting and/or sufficiently retaining adolescents living with HIV without the ability to meet multiple levels of needs within a continuum of care model (Bettencourt et al., 1998; Bourdon, Tierney, Huba, Lothrop, Melchior, Betru, & Compoc, 1998; Huba & Melchior, 1998; Schneir et al., 1998). This does not need to be comprehensively available within one service setting, but must be anticipated by an agency, which then must establish linkages across agencies to meet the needs of these youth. Adolescents living with HIV who received care at LSYC would not have been admitted to substance abuse treatment and would have dropped out if admitted. These clients continued their drug use while maintaining themselves in the community; however, there were substantial clinical improvements among these youth even though they continued using drugs, and there did appear to be reductions in some substances.

Assessing the success of a continuum of care model must be measured by monitoring the health and quality of life outcomes for the system's clients. This may be accomplished by collecting and analyzing individual and collective client data regarding physical and mental health, stability of life, and degree of progress toward meeting individual needs (i.e., accomplishing personal goals). It will also be important to monitor the rates of client service utilization, retention, successful referrals, and adherence to treatment regimens.

The case studies presented in this paper highlight the need for long-term residential care for disabled HIV-seropositive youth. Youth's life histories indicated the absence of family support over many years; in fact, the family has typically been the source of the stressors and abuse experienced by the youth. Youth with multiple problems, i.e., those comorbid for substance use and mental health disorders, are only likely to be treated effectively in social service settings that are integrated so that care is comprehensive, coordinated, and seamless. In Australia, providers of community-based services to homeless youth are legally responsible to ensure that youth have a placement and long-term, comprehensive care (Hillier, Matthews, & Dempsey, 1997). In the United States, community-based providers do not have similar responsibilities nor guaranteed, ongoing funding to provide such services. Only a few community-based agencies have been able to patch together the comprehensive, multi-level services provided by LSYC. Without such comprehensive services, it is likely that the HIV-seropositive youth would die in circumstances of continued sex bartering and daily drug use. In 1994, three HIV-positive youth died in different circumstances: one went through a window from an upper floor; one died alone at night in assisted housing, and one died in a drug bust gone sour. By providing the stable housing, LSYC has created the possibility that the youth may die surrounded by friends and caretakers after having chosen a legacy and, perhaps, having even planned their funeral. Housing provides youth the choice not to stand on a street corner to turn a trick (especially on a rainy night). This is a fundamental change that provides stability in survival needs. Receiving antiretrovirals, now a basic component of survival for the seropositive, is also only possible in this context.

Only a few youth in each of our urban, inner cities need long-term housing and comprehensive care. Yet, for those few, the failure to provide such care violates the UN Children's Bill of Rights. It is important that we replicate such care for those who need it.

REFERENCES

American Psychiatric Association. (1998). *Diagnostic and statistical manual of mental disorders*. Washington, D.C.: Author.

Archer, S. L. (1989). The status of identity: Reflections on the need for intervention. Special Issue: Adolescent identity. An appraisal of health and intervention. *Journal of Adolescence, 12* (4), 345-359.

Bettencourt, T., Hodgins, A., Huba, G. J., & Pickett, G. (1998). Bay Area Young

Positives: A model of a youth-based approach to HIV/AIDS services. *Journal of Adolescent Health, 23* (Suppl.), S28-36.

Bourdon, B., Tierney, S., Huba, G. J., Lothrop, J., Melchior, L. A., Betru, R., & Compoc, K. (1998). Health Initiatives for Youth: A model of youth/adult partnership approach to HIV/AIDS services. *Journal of Adolescent Health, 23* (Suppl.), S71-82.

Bowler, S., Sheon, A. R., D'Angelo, L. J., & Vermund, S. H. (1992). HIV and AIDS among adolescents in the United States: Increasing risk in the 1990s. *Journal of Adolescence, 15,* 345-371.

Centers for Disease Control and Prevention. (1998a). *HIV/AIDS Surveillance Report: U.S. HIV and AIDS cases reported through June 1998, 10* (1), 1-40.

Centers for Disease Control and Prevention. (1998b). *Update: Young people at risk-epidemic shifts further toward young women and minorities.* Atlanta, GA: Author.

Centers for Disease Control and Prevention. (1998c). HIV infection in disadvantaged out-of-school youth: Prevalence for U.S. job corps entrants, 1990 through 1996. *Journal of Acquired Immune Deficiency Syndromes and Human Retrovirology, 19* (1).

Children's Defense Fund. (1988). *A children's defense budget FY 1989: An analysis of our nation's investment in children.* Washington, DC: Author.

Conviser, R. (1993). *Serving young people at risk for HIV infection: Case studies of adolescent-focused HIV prevention and service delivery programs.* Newark, NJ: National Pediatric HIV Resource Center.

D'Angelo, L. J. (1991, October 1). *A longitudinal study of HIV infection in urban adolescents.* Presented at the Intersciences Conference on Antimicrobal Agents and Chemotherapy, Chicago, IL.

D'Angelo, L. J., Getson, P. R., Luban, N. L. C., & Gayle, H. D. (1991). Human immunodeficiency virus (HIV) in urban adolescents. *Pediatrics, 88,* 982-986.

English, A. (1995). The HIV challenge: Prevention education for young people. In M. Quackenbush & M. Nelson (Eds., 2nd ed.), *Adolescents and HIV: Legal and ethical questions* (pp. 259-285).

Gayle, H. D., & D'Angelo, L. J. (1991). Epidemiology of acquired immunodeficiency syndrome and human immunodeficiency virus infection in adolescents. *Pediatric Infectious Disease Journal, 10* (4), 322-328.

Glaser, R., & Kiecolt-Glaser, J. K. (1987). Stress-associated depression in cellular immunity: Implications for acquired immune deficiency syndrome (AIDS). *Brain, Behavior & Immunity, 2* (2), 117-112.

Gwadz, M., De Vogli, R., Rotheram-Borus, M. J., Diaz, M. M., Cisek, T., James, N. B., & Tottenham, N. (in press). Behavioral practices regarding combination therapies for HIV/AIDS. *Journal of Sex Education and Therapy.*

Hein, K. (1989). AIDS in adolescence: Exploring the challenge. *Journal of Adolescent Health care, 10* (Suppl.), S10-35.

Hillier, L., Matthews, L., & Dempsey, D. (1997). *A low priority in a hierarchy of needs: A profile of the sexual health of young homeless people in Australia.* Carlton South, Victoria, Australia: National Centre in HIV Social Research: Program in Youth/General Population.

Horwitz, R. I., & Horwitz, S. M. (1993). Adherence to treatment and health outcomes. *Archives of Internal Medicine, 153,* 1863-1868.

Huba, G. J., & Melchior, L. A. (1998). A model for adolescent-targeted HIV/AIDS services: Conclusions from 10 adolescent-targeted projects funded by the Special Projects of National Significance Program of the Health Resources and Services Administration. *Journal of Adolescent Health, 23* (Suppl.), S11-27.

Izard, C. E., Kagan. J., & Zajonc, R. B. (1984). *Emotions, Cognition & Behavior.* New York: Cambridge University Press.

Karon, J. M., Rosenberg, P. S., McQuillan, G., Khare, M., Gwinn, M., & Peterson L. R. (1996). Prevalence of HIV infection in the United States, 1984 to 1992. *JAMA, 276,* 126.

Kemeny, M. E. (1994). Stressful events, psychological responses, and progression of HIV infection. In R. Glaser & J. K. Kiecolt-Glaser (Eds.), *Handbook of human stress and immunity* (pp. 245-266). San Diego, CA: Academic Press, Inc.

Lange, J. M. (1995). Current HIV clinical trial design issues. *Journal of Acquired Immune Deficiency Syndromes and Human Retrovirology, 10* (Suppl. 1), S47-51.

Larkin Street Youth Center. (1998a). Profile of Programs. San Francisco, CA: Author.

Larkin Street Youth Center. (1998b). Title IV Adolescent Services Application, Draft, June 18. San Francisco, CA: Author.

Maslow, A. (1987). *Motivation and personality* (3rd ed.). New York: Harper & Row.

Matlin, M. (1983). *Cognition.* New York: The Dryden Press.

Morris, M., Zavisca, J., & Dean, L. (1995). Social and sexual networks: Their role in the spread of HIV/AIDS among young gay men. *AIDS Education and Prevention, 7* (Suppl.), 24-35.

Moss, G. B., Clemetson, D., D'Costa, L., Plummer, F. A., Ndinya-Achola, J. O., Reilly, M., Holmes, K. K., Piot, P., Maitha, G. M., Hillier, S. L. et al. (1991). Association of cervical ectopy with heterosexual transmission of Human Immune Deficiency Virus: Results of a study of couples in Nairobi, Kenya. *Journal of Infectious Diseases, 164,* 588-591.

Nelson, H. (1996). Protease inhibitors show promise in HIV infection. *Lancet, 347* (8998), 383.

O'Brien, M. K., Petrie, K., & Raeburn, J. (1992). Adherence to medication regimens: Updating a complex medical issue. *Medical Care Review, 49* (4), 435-454.

Rotheram-Borus, M. J., Feldman, J., Rosario, M., & Dunne, E. (1994). Preventing HIV among runaways: Victims and victimization. In R. DiClemente & J. Peterson (Eds.), *Preventing AIDS: Theories and methods of behavioral interventions* (pp. 175-188). New York: Plenum Press.

Rotheram-Borus, M. J., Murphy, D. A., Coleman, C. L., Kennedy, M., Reid, H. M., Cline, T. R., Birnbaum, J. M., Futterman, D., Levin, L., Schneir, A., Chabon, B., O'Keefe, Z., & Kipke, M. (1997). Risk acts, healthcare, and medical adherence among HIV-positive youths in care over time. *AIDS and Behavior, 1,* 43-52.

Rotheram-Borus, M. J., Murphy, D. A., Fernandez, M. I., & Srinivasan, S. (1998). A brief HIV intervention for adolescents and young adults. *American Journal of Orthopsychiatry, 68,* 553-564.

San Francisco AIDS Foundation. (1998, January). Adherence and the HIV community. *Bulletin of Experimental Treatment for AIDS.*

Schlebusch, L., & Cassidy, M. J. (1995). Stress, social support and biopsychosocial dynamics in HIV/AIDS. Special focus: Psychological aspects of HIV/AIDS. *South African Journal of Psychology, 25* (1), 27-30.

Schneir, A., Kipke, M. D., Melchior, L. A., & Huba, G. J. (1998). Childrens Hospital Los Angeles: A model of integrated care for HIV-positive and very high-risk youth. *Journal of Adolescent Health, 23* (Suppl.), S59-70.

Shalwitz, J. C., Goulart, M., Dunnigan, K., & Flannery, D. (1990). *Prevalence of sexually transmitted diseases (STD) and HIV in a homeless youth medical clinic in San Francisco.* Abstracts of the Sixth International Conference on AIDS, San Francisco, CA (Vol. 3, pp. 231, No. S.C.571).

St. Louis, M. E., Conway, G. A., Hayman, C. R., Miller, C., Petersen, L. R., & Dondero, T. J. (1991). Human immunodeficiency virus infection in disadvantaged adolescents: Findings from the U.S. Job Corps. *JAMA, 266,* 2387-2391.

Stricof, R. L., Novick, L. F., & Kennedy, J. T. (1990). *HIV-1 seroprevalence in facilities for runaway and homeless adolescents in four states: Florida, Texas, Louisiana, and New York.* Abstract presented at the Sixth International Conference on AIDS, San Francisco, CA (Abstract No. F.C.47).

Stricof, R. L., Kennedy, J. T., Nattell, T. C., Weisfuse, I. B., & Novick, L. (1991). HIV seroprevalence in a facility for minority and homeless adolescents. *American Journal of Public Health, 81* (Suppl.) 50-53.

UNAIDS Joint United Nations Programme on HIV/AIDS. (1998). *AIDS epidemic update: December 1998.* Available on the Web at http://www.who.int/emc-hiv/. Author.

U.S. Conference of Mayors. (1987). *The continued growth of hunger, homelessness and poverty in America's cities in 1986.* Washington, DC: Author.

Yurgelun-Todd, D. A. (1998, June 11). *Functional MRI studies of adolescents: Frontal temporal changes.* Presented at the Brain and Psyche Seminar, Whitehead Institute for Biomedical Research, Cambridge, MA.

Drug and Alcohol Use Among Boston's Haitian Community: A Hidden Problem Unveiled by CCHER's Enhanced Innovative Case Management Program

Eustache Jean-Louis, MD, MPH
Janine Walker, MPH
Guy Apollon, MD, LCSW
Joel Piton, MD
M. Berthonia Antoine
Alfred Mombeleur
Marc Thelismond
Nicole César

SUMMARY. This article discusses the Enhanced Innovative Case Management Program of CCHER, Inc., a community-based agency

Eustache Jean-Louis, Janine Walker, Guy Apollon, Joel Piton, M. Berthonia Antoine, Alfred Mombeleur, Marc Thelismond, and Nicole César are affiliated with The Center for Community Health Education and Research, Dorchester, MA.

Address correspondence to: Eustache Jean-Louis, MD, MPH, Center for Community Health Education and Research, Haitian Community AIDS Outreach Project, 420 Washington Street, Dorchester, MA 02124 (E-mail: ccherhap@ccher.org).

This work was supported in part by the Health Resources and Services Administration (HRSA), HIV/AIDS Bureau (HAB), Special Projects of National Significance (SPNS) Grant No. BRU 900123-05. This publication's contents are solely the responsibility of the authors and do not necessarily represent the official view of the funding agency.

[Haworth co-indexing entry note]: "Drug and Alcohol Use Among Boston's Haitian Community: A Hidden Problem Unveiled by CCHER's Enhanced Innovative Case Management Program." Jean-Louis, Eustache et al. Co-published simultaneously in *Drugs & Society* (The Haworth Press, Inc.) Vol. 16, No. 1/2, 2000, pp. 107-122; and: *Evaluating HIV/AIDS Treatment Programs: Innovative Methods and Findings* (ed: G. J. Huba et al.) The Haworth Press, Inc., 2000, pp. 107-122. Single or multiple copies of this article are available for a fee from The Haworth Document Delivery Service [1-800-342-9678, 9:00 a.m. - 5:00 p.m. (EST). E-mail address: getinfo@haworthpressinc.com].

serving Boston's immigrant Haitian population living with HIV/AIDS. A psychosocial educational counseling program of 25 topics was created to address psychosocial needs of Haitian HIV consumers. Counseling sessions are one-to-one, in Haitian Creole. A pre-post evaluation design assesses the effectiveness of the curriculum in relation to the objectives of the project. The project has allowed CCHER to identify complex substance abuse issues and as a result has enabled the agency to address substance abuse among Haitians and plan culturally appropriate educational, outreach, and counseling strategies for Haitian substance abusers and community members. *[Article copies available for a fee from The Haworth Document Delivery Service: 1-800-342-9678. E-mail address: <getinfo@haworthpressinc.com> Website: <http://www.HaworthPress. com>]*

KEYWORDS. Haitian, HIV/AIDS, substance abuse, immigrants, cultural competence, Haitian Creole, Psychosocial Educational Counseling (PEC), health beliefs, cross-cutting data

INTRODUCTION

The combined impact of alcohol and drug use causes multiple diseases and is costly to our healthcare system (Fox, Merrill, Chang, & Califana, 1995). Studies of the broad impact of alcohol and drug use on different ethnic groups are well documented in the epidemiological literature. Currently, however, there is very little information available in the literature related to substance abuse among Haitians living here in the U.S. Data on Haitians, if existing at all, is scant and is oftentimes incorporated into data on African Americans, thereby providing little specific information on this ethnic community. The Center for Community Health, Education and Research, Inc. (CCHER), a community-based organization operated by Haitian professionals and located in the heart of Boston's Haitian community, has provided culturally competent health and social services to the local Haitian community and to Haitians living with HIV since 1987. CCHER has provided a psychosocial educational counseling program (PEC) to Haitians living with HIV through funding from the Health Resources and Services Administration's (HRSA) Special Projects of National Significance (SPNS). This tested model of intervention has allowed CCHER counselors to identify important issues in consumers' lives that may otherwise remain veiled in secrecy, such as substance abuse and addiction. This paper will describe how the SPNS-funded psychosocial educational counseling model for Haitians has been a catalyst in enabling CCHER to identify substance abuse and addiction within the community; how CCHER has begun the early stages of identifying, understanding, and clearly defining the needs of the Haitian community in relation to substance abuse and addiction; and how, as a result, CCHER has begun implementing culturally competent services targeted at Haitian substance abusers and their families.

Background

The second half of the twentieth century has seen large numbers of Haitians emigrating to the United States. Fleeing a fragile and oftentimes brutal political system, tremendous poverty, and other poor social conditions, Haitians seek a better life here in the U.S. While increasing numbers of Haitians had begun to arrive in the 1950s and early 1960s, the more decisive phase of Haitian migration began in the late 1970s. During this later phase, very poor Haitians from the rural peasant culture endured dangerous and oftentimes tragic journeys by sea to reach the shores of Southern Florida (Preeg, 1996). Haitian immigrants here in the U.S. come from all sectors of Haitian society, varying in social class, skin color, level of education, religious beliefs, language preference, and geographical place of origin (Zephir, 1996).

Upon their arrival into North America, Haitians have settled within the cities of Montreal, Miami, Chicago, Boston, and most prominently, in New York City. There are no precise figures on the number of U.S. residents of Haitian origin; estimates obviously fail to take into account a large number of undocumented entrants. The best estimates indicate that there are about 1 million Haitians or Haitian-Americans here in the United States (Preeg, 1996). Boston's Haitian community, one of the larger in the U.S., is one of the city's fastest growing ethnic communities. An estimated 45,000 Haitian immigrants have settled into the city of Boston, with some statewide estimates as high as 75,000 (MDPH, 1998).

The HIV Epidemic in the Haitian Community

Miller (1984) notes that of the diseases that have affected the Haitian community both here and in the homeland, none seems to have had greater consequences than AIDS. In the early 1980s, Haitians were the only ethnic group ever singled out within the U.S. as an at-risk group for AIDS. This served to further increase the stigma surrounding the disease and caused fear and discrimination towards the Haitian community. Haitians in the U.S. were seen as "AIDS carriers"; many lost jobs and housing due to the hysteria created by this labeling of the Haitian community (Farmer, 1992). In the late 1980s, an FDA regulation excluded Haitians from donating blood, a ban that was eagerly challenged by Haitian community leaders throughout the U.S. This ban was later repealed.

In addition to being stigmatized by the outside community, HIV infected Haitians suffer their own intra-community stigmatization which often results from strong moral ideals rooted firmly in religion. This ideology yields explanations for diseases that are often based on immoral behaviors. Culturally-based conceptions of disease also contribute to intra-community stigma and can play a major role in diminishing Haitians' utilization of existing services. As with other immigrant groups, the social, cultural, and economic context of their lives will influence their decisions to use formal healthcare (Leclere, Jensen, & Biddlecom, 1994). Many Haitians, whether or not they are familiar with biochemical concepts and medical treatment, may not always respond immediately to concepts of the American medical system. Traditionally they do not seek medical attention until late in the course of their illness; self-treatment is common, and hospitals tend to be regarded as a final resource center for solving medical problems (Laguerre, 1981). Angel and Guarnaccia (1989) have asserted that medical need is determined not only by the presence of physical disease but also, in part, by the cultural perception of illness. For example, Haitians may attribute being infected with HIV or drug addiction to supernatural causes. Some Haitians believe that diseases are sent by the gods, and must therefore be fatalistically accepted. Others believe diseases have been induced through sorcery, as punishment for past behaviors. "God will take care of it" is a popular expression used to deny acceptance of a disease diagnosis or to explain Haitians' reluctance to seek medical attention. These cultural factors are deeply imbedded in the Haitian psyche and over time influence decisions about health and contribute to morbidity within the community. They also present complex challenges for health and social service providers involved in the care of the Haitian consumer.

CCHER's Special Project of National Significance

CCHER's Enhanced Innovative Case Management Program (EICMP) was created to provide HIV-positive Haitian consumers with the opportunity to discuss, in-depth and in Haitian Creole, the psychosocial issues and risk reduction challenges that they may face as they live with their HIV/AIDS. Over the course of the five year project, CCHER developed and implemented a Psychosocial Educational Counseling (PEC) curriculum for Haitian HIV consumers that addressed coping strategies, consumer's sense of well being, the healthcare system, concepts of health and illness, and prevention/risk reduction associated with HIV transmission. The program was created to: (1) increase consumers' knowledge of how to prevent HIV transmissions; (2) increase consumers' adherence to treatment; (3) improve consumers' utilization of health and social services; (4) increase consumers' satisfaction with case management services and other services received; (5) reduce risk behaviors; and (6) improve consumers' sense of well being.

The Psychosocial Educational Counseling Curriculum

CCHER's Psychosocial Educational Counseling (PEC) Curriculum consists of 25 psychosocial topics relevant to the Haitian HIV consumer (see

Table 1). PEC is administered one-to-one between a consumer and a Haitian counselor, in Haitian Creole. The curriculum is a flexible, consumer-centered model that is based on nonjudgmental, active listening and the "unconditional faith that consumers, if given the right tools and a culturally competent counselor, over time, can take charge of events that affect their lives." The content of consumer-counselor interactions and the timing and manner in which topics are presented are heavily dependent on the counselor's clinical judgment. While the relationship between counselor and consumer is central in any therapeutic interaction, particular care is required with this population. Suspicion of public institutions, reluctance to receive what may be perceived as "charity," fear due to immigration status, stigma, negative experiences with healthcare providers, and the taboos surrounding sex and death all make the initial bridges between consumer and counselor particularly fragile.

Program Design and Implementation

A pre-post questionnaire design was created to assess the effectiveness of the counseling intervention. The program is divided into four phases: During phases one and two, consumers become acclimated to the program, sign an informed consent form, and complete baseline data. During phase three, consumers receive the one-to-one counseling sessions with their counselors. Once they have completed the 25 topic curriculum, they undergo a six month 'assimilation period' in which they do not have formal counseling with their CCHER counselor, but they do continue to receive other services from the agency. Six months after their completion of the counseling curriculum, they are followed up and questionnaires are re-administered, along with an exit interview. The local project evaluation combined the use of cross-cutting data collection modules for the overall cooperative agreement (Huba, Melchior, Brown, & Larson, 2000) with CCHER's own in-house questionnaires. CCHER designed two culturally relevant questionnaires that capture knowledge, attitudes, beliefs and behaviors of enrollees. The local evaluation also utilized qualitative data in the form of focus groups, discussions with providers, and discussions with counselors. Selection of appropriate data collection instruments and creation of CCHER questionnaires were designed to assess, over time, the impact the counseling program has had on consumers related to the six evaluation criteria noted above.

Consumers began enrolling into the project in late 1995. To date, 67 Haitian adults living with HIV/AIDS have been enrolled into the project, 38 females and 29 males. Consumers range in age from 19 to 63 years old. At this time, demographic characteristics are available for 49 enrollees. All 49 consumers listed Creole as their primary language. Ninety-two percent (92%) self-identified their sexual orientation as heterosexual. Eighteen percent (18%) described themselves as employed part-time or full-time. Thirty-nine percent (39%) of this sample described themselves as having no source of income. Questions about

TABLE 1. Psychosocial Educational Counseling Curriculum

Topic 1: Alcohol Use and Abuse

Topic 2: Substance Abuse and HIV/AIDS Among Haitians

Topic 3: Mental Health

Topic 4: HIV Pre-Test Counseling

Topic 5: HIV Post-Test Counseling

Topic 6: Individual Counseling and Therapy

Topic 7: Guardianship for Haitian Parents Living with HIV/AIDS

Topic 8: Domestic Violence and the HIV Connection

Topic 9: Barriers to Care for HIV+ Haitians

Topic 10: Sexuality and Self-Identity

Topic 11: Legal Problems

Topic 12: HIV Disclosure

Topic 13: Treatment Adherence

Topic 14: Public Assistance

Topic 15: Family Planning

Topic 16: Dating, Sex, and HIV

Topic 17: Concepts of Health and Illness

Topic 18: Emotions and Emotional Problems Related to HIV/AIDS

Topic 19: HIV/AIDS as a Chronic Health Problem

Topic 20: Managing Stages of HIV Disease

Topic 21: Haitian Women Living with HIV/AIDS

Topic 22: Haitian Men Living with HIV/AIDS

Topic 23: Parents of Haitian Adolescents with HIV

Topic 24: Seniors and HIV/AIDS

Topic 25: Tuberculosis and HIV/AIDS Among Haitians

behaviors in relation to HIV/AIDS are elicited from consumers on this questionnaire. Thirty-one percent (31%) of consumers cited an inferred alcohol problem as occurring 'currently' (last 30 days) or 'ever' (has occurred, but not in last 30 days). Three of these individuals were females. Six percent (6%) listed crack use as 'current' or 'ever.' These were all males. Twelve percent (12%) listed other illicit drug use as 'current' or 'ever.' One of these was female. One male indicated that he had 'ever' used injection drugs and had shared needles.

The SPNS Project: Linking HIV and Substance Abuse

The notion of counseling is relatively new and unfamiliar to some Haitians; for most, discussing their sexual activity and other intimate, personal information with a stranger or even a provider is a new phenomenon that they are generally unaccustomed to. For those consumers that are able to establish a sense of comfort and a level of trust with their CCHER counselors, the SPNS counseling program can allow them to unload tremendous psychosocial burdens, far more complex than often anticipated. Consider the following case illustration:

This is a case of a thirty-five year old Haitian woman with a history of being raped in Haiti as a child, sexual promiscuity since age 11, attempted suicide, and domestic abuse in her life. She had moved to Boston in the early 1990s from New York after her HIV diagnosis incited tremendous blame and stigma from her family. Her family blamed her for her behaviors, and her HIV diagnosis was seen as her punishment from God for her dirty behaviors and attitudes. She became dependent on alcohol, although she never considered that she might be addicted. Her provider offered help to get her in touch with a Haitian counselor who could talk to her. Initially, she refused without hesitation; she did not want to get involved with Haitian providers. She held a professional position in the community and wanted to protect her reputation and identity. After hearing a CCHER Haitian counselor speak at a mental health clinic, she got in touch with the counselor and made an appointment to speak with her. The CCHER counselor began to make home visits to the woman and slowly began to establish a relationship with her. She began to trust her counselor and enrolled in the CCHER SPNS program. After a lengthy process of engaging in frank discussions with her counselor on the psychosocial educational counseling topics, the woman revealed that she was addicted to alcohol, marijuana and sleeping pills. The counselor reports that the woman felt a tremendous burden lifted off of her after she was able to disclose her addictions. The counselor was able to work with her on some of her issues as the PEC curriculum continued. This facilitated, among other things, a referral for detox treatment.

As with the case of this particular woman, consumers oftentimes come to the program with tremendous psychosocial burdens. They have seldom been given the appropriate milieu to discuss these burdens in a linguistically and culturally appropriate manner. The PEC sessions not only meet the linguistic needs of this population, they give the consumer the opportunity of talking with a Haitian professional who has knowledge of the norms, the values and the context of their everyday lives in relation to sense of family and community, religion, health and illness beliefs and behaviors, histories, and experiences in their homeland of Haiti. In CCHER's model, it is the Haitian professional who has a tremendous sense of how and what the Haitian consumer understands and as such can deliver services in a culturally competent approach.

Substance Abuse in the Haitian Community

During its many years of working with Haitians amidst the HIV epidemic, CCHER has often encountered Haitians with HIV who were using cocaine, marijuana, and/or alcohol. Yet because of the high rates of heterosexual HIV transmission among Haitians and the low rates of AIDS diagnosed as a result of IDU, establishing a link between alcohol and illicit drug use and HIV transmission was never a top priority. Just four percent of the reported 630 cases of AIDS among Massachusetts Haitians are categorized as transmission through injecting drug use (MDPH AIDS Surveillance Bureau, January 1999). This low rate of reported IDU as a risk factor is consistent with other studies on Haitians and HIV transmission (Viera, Frank, Spira, & Landesman 1983; Adrien, Boivin, Tousignant, & Hankins, 1990). Because of the complex histories of substance abuse and addiction issues that became evident among some of the SPNS project enrollees, it became necessary to begin a dialogue at CCHER about substance abuse and bring it to the forefront of the agency's programming. Alcohol and drug abuse are often topics that remain hidden among many Haitians and not talked about, due to the sense of shame it often brings upon those in the community. In Haiti, alcohol is very common at social functions. There is very little focus on alcohol and drug prevention programs; and many Haitians are unfamiliar with therapy and counseling. Nor are there ample treatment facilities in Haiti for those that are fighting the disease of addiction. "Addiction" is not a concept easily understood among many Haitians. Alcohol and drug abuse is commonly not regarded as an illness for which one needs to seek professional attention. Alcohol and drug use is seen as something that can be handled by the individual. The Haitian may see it only as a problem when one hits 'rock bottom,' i.e., when one has been rejected by family, is now living on the street, is involved in domestic violence, is involved in drug trafficking or the court system, can't hold a job, and is unclean and unkempt. A common Creole term related to this is referred to as *"de pye pran nan yon sél grenn soulye"* or *"having two feet in one shoe,"* the notion of being trapped and having no place to go.

Many Haitians may believe that this condition is not an emotional or medical problem. This condition is not a coincidence; it is, rather, *li dejwe,* a condition sent as a curse due to the envy and jealousy of a girlfriend or boyfriend. *Li dejwe* is believed to be a curse that prohibits the person from reaching their full potential. This notion of sickness being 'sent' incorporates traditional health and illness beliefs of Haitians and has been well documented (Martin, Rissmiller, & Beal, 1995; Laguerre, 1984). At this point, families may offer their help to the person, or simply reject the substance abuser. Help, within the framework of the Haitian family member or friend, is not in the form of assisting the person in seeking medical or psychological treatment, but may instead be in the form of traditional folk detoxification treatments to cleanse the body. A CCHER counselor gave an example of one such mixture:

One creates a mixture consisting of the sweat of a horse, leaves, resin oil and a large quantity of tobacco leaves and it is drunk. This mixture acts as a cleanser for the body to purge it of alcohol. This may cause a person to become violently ill, and may even result in death. Once a Haitian has drunk this, any subsequent consumption of alcohol will result in this violent purging effect, not allowing the person to absorb any more alcohol, thereby effectively 'curing' the person.

Lack of an Adequate Profile on Haitian Substance Abusers

While the literature provides ample analysis of substance abuse among minority and immigrant communities here in the United States, it is mainly limited to those of Hispanic, African American, Asian, and Native American origin (Rebach, 1992). To our knowledge, virtually nothing in the literature exists that specifically explores Haitians and Haitian Americans as a separate entity and addresses factors contributing to, the treatment for, or the prevention of substance abuse. Much of the data collected nationwide tends to lump most black ethnic minorities into the category of 'Black' rather than taking into account national origin and the specific cultural and linguistic characteristics of individual groups. Zephir (1996) commented that in New York, Caribbean immigrants are placed within two categories: 'Black' and 'Hispanic.' Laguerre (1981) noted that most statistical studies merge Haitians with other American Blacks. This grouping of all ethnic minorities on the basis of skin color fails to take into account the cultural influences and nuances that can have critical implications for substance abuse education, prevention and treatment for the Haitian community. Watson, Mattera, Morales, Kunitz, and Lynch (1985), in their study of alcohol use among Black and Haitian migrant agricultural workers in Western New York, noted that "little is known about Haitian drinking behavior in the United States, or even in Haiti" (p. 406). Given this dearth of information, CCHER is learning first hand from an intracommunity perspective about the behaviors, the beliefs, the cultural influences, and the needs of the Haitian community in relation to substance abuse and addiction.

Haitians in the city of Boston, as in the other cities where they have settled, remain a tightly knit community both geographically and socially. Most continue to maintain their strong cultural identities in association with religion, food, music, art, language, and ties to the homeland. In her sociological portrait of Haitian immigrants, Zephir (1996) asserted that most Haitians do not assimilate with other native or immigrant communities here in the U.S., and therefore, maintain themselves as a distinct ethnic group in the United States. As such, this cultural uniqueness cannot be captured in any of the existing literature of drug and alcohol abuse among minority groups in the United States. Rebach (1992), in his research on alcohol and drug use among American minorities, looked at 4 ethnic groups here in the U.S.: African American, Hispanic, Asian, and Native Americans. While the distinct cultural identity of the Haitian community does not neatly "fit" into any one of the groups in Rebach's analysis, generalizations about the four groups as a whole in many ways pertain to the Haitian community that CCHER is serving, and have important implications for culturally competent programming within the agency.

Rebach (1992) asserts that sociocultural influences can play a role in substance abuse. Conflict between the dominant culture and various minority cultures may be an underlying causative factor in substance use. Alcohol use may be seen as an attempt to cope with stress from unemployment, poverty, inadequate housing, all which may result from poor integration into the economic opportunity structure. Indeed, for many Haitians struggling in a new land, the cultural and linguistic barriers can often be overwhelming. As newcomers, these immigrants face seemingly insurmountable barriers in many areas, including language, literacy, cultural adaptation, immigration status, discrimination, and socioeconomic survival. These vulnerabilities, the foundation for which the SPNS Psychosocial Educational Counseling Curriculum was created, can no doubt lead to tremendous environmental stressors, of which alcohol and substance use can sometimes be a response.

Rebach also notes that minority persons are less likely to seek treatment and less likely to complete treatment once begun. Cultural values may influence treatment. Many treatment programs lack an understanding of and sensitivity to ethnic cultures. This understanding and sensitivity is necessary to be effective with consumers. The most frequent suggestion to remedy the lack of cultural sensitivity is that programs be staffed by members similar in ethnicity to those being served. Given the basic assertions of the minority experience in America and its relationship to substance abuse, it is easy to understand that a community with what Zephir (1996) refers to as "triple minority status"–foreign, black, and non-English speaking–needs specifically tailored tools and culturally competent approaches towards effective substance abuse services.

Specific Substance Abuse Prevention Strategies

CCHER Substance Abuse staff reported that many Haitians don't utilize the substance abuse services available to them within the city. As a result, CCHER's newly created substance abuse department has been extremely busy in developing programming to meet the needs of the local Haitian community. Culturally competent approaches have begun to be developed and continue to be refined within several areas.

METHODS

Three specific methods of intervention were identified as being particularly appropriate to the community. These were: outreach and education, community level training, and case management and advocacy. These interventions will be summarized below.

Outreach and education. The first method of intervention is outreaching and educating the general community. CCHER has found, over the years, that radio is one of the most effective outlets for outreaching to the Haitian community. Radio is a very popular information medium among Haitians in Haiti as well as here in the U.S. Multiple Haitian radio projects in the Boston area provide Haitians with a vital link to their homeland; they also provide Boston's Haitian community with valuable health and educational information in Haitian Creole. As part of its outreach and educational initiatives, CCHER's substance abuse department conducts monthly radio segments to raise awareness on drugs and addiction, the ramifications of drug abuse on individuals and families, and the link between substance abuse, sexual behavior, and HIV. Those listening to the popular radio program are allowed to call into the program for questions and discussion. Outreach and education activities also include CCHER Substance Abuse staff conducting informational sessions on "HIV and the Substance Abuse Connection" within the community at local churches, community organizations, and schools. These sessions focus on how the use of alcohol and drugs can influence decision-making about sexual behaviors, leading to high-risk sexual activity.

Community-level training and dissemination. A second intervention method is a peer-based model. A culturally competent educational and training approach is providing Haitians in the community critical information about substance abuse, addiction, and the link to HIV. Similar to a highly successful HIV "Volunteer Health Educators" (VHE) educational model that already exists here at CCHER, the "Alcohol and Other Drugs Program" is a 3-week training program conducted in Haitian Creole. The training program is designed to bring to those identified to be volunteer health educators the latest information about drug use and addiction. It introduces community members, affected family members, and consumers to the notion of addiction, the signs and symptoms of alcoholism and drug addiction, and available community resources. It also addresses how addiction and crime can be linked and can lead to legal ramifications such as jail, immigration dilemmas, and even deportation. Culturally appropriate questionnaires have been created to assess community participants' knowledge, attitudes, and beliefs about drugs and addiction. Recruited participants for the program receive approximately 32 hours of didactic instructions and skills-based activities. See Table 2 for the Alcohol and Other Drugs Program Curriculum.

Participants are trained to become volunteer health educators to disseminate the information to their community. Once participants have completed the program, they must present what they have learned to friends and family within a home-presentation setting. These smaller intimate gatherings that

TABLE 2. "Alcohol and Other Drug Program" Training Curriculum

Social Implications of Alcohol and Other Drugs and the HIV Connection

Concepts of Health and Disease: How Haitians Understand Addiction

Human Services in the U.S.

Impact of Haitian Culture on Our Health: Barriers vs. Benefits

HIV/AIDS: Biological and Mental Health Aspects

STDs: Cause and Effect, Symptoms, Signs and Treatments

Drug Paraphernalia: What Are They, What Do They Look Like?

Biological Impact of Alcohol and Other Drugs on the Brain and Human Body

Addiction and Treatment Implications

Clinical Aspects and Theories for Inpatient Treatment

Causes and Effects of Addiction, Homelessness

Outpatient Treatment: How It Works, and for Whom

Psychosocial Counseling Therapy: Healing Methods

Differences in Sexual Lifestyles in Connection with HIV/AIDS, Alcohol and Other Drugs

Site Visit to Recovery Home for Addicts and Their Families

Experiences and Benefits of Recovery by Consumers

Role of Spirituality in Addiction and Chronic Illness

participants conduct allow for frank discussion about substance abuse and its implications in a comfortable, non-threatening atmosphere among Haitians in the community. Five training programs have thus far taken place, training a total of 84 Haitian adults and older teens. These 84 participants have in turn reached over 420 Haitians within the community to spread the word about addiction and treatment.

Case management/advocacy. The third method of intervention is a consumer-centered model of case management and advocacy, providing services to active substance abusers, those in recovery, and their families. These services are in the early stages of development. Through self-referral, street outreach, hospital referral, and court referrals, consumers are linked with one of two CCHER Haitian outreach workers/substance abuse specialists. These staff work with consumers and their families providing informal counseling, education, crisis intervention, relapse prevention, translation, advocacy, and accompaniment. Staff work to ultimately guide the consumer towards drug-free living.

Lessons Being Learned

When the Substance Abuse program began in the Fall of 1997 as a small pilot project, CCHER anticipated serving just over 20 substance abusing Haitians within the community. Already in the first eighteen months of the project,

45 consumers are receiving case management/advocacy services from CCHER staff. CCHER currently serves 33 males and 12 females and works with their families as well. Six of these were enrolled in the SPNS program and then became involved in the substance abuse programming. Many consumers are addicted to a combination of alcohol and drugs; all of these consumers admit to sniffing and smoking cocaine. None report injecting drug use. Most consumers are between the ages of 20 and 49, while one male is over age 50. Seven of these consumers are HIV-positive; many others have yet to test. Fifteen consumers have records with the law, with four consumers facing deportation in the near future. Seven consumers are illiterate.

CCHER staff are finding that some who are receiving services are triple-diagnosed: they are living with HIV, suffer from addiction, and have tremendous mental health needs. The complex issues that consumers have presented are, CCHER believes, just the tip of the iceberg in what has evolved to be a challenging task of addressing the substance abuse needs of the Haitian community. CCHER Substance Abuse staff have begun to see critical areas in which vital services are needed for Haitians:

Homelessness is a common problem among many substance abusers seeking services at CCHER; several consumers are living in shelters or living on the streets. It is also very common for many consumers to bounce around from one residence to another, seeking temporary shelter on an available bed, couch or floor space of a friend or family member. This instability prevents many from becoming drug-free and prevents many from maintaining a drug-free existence if they are in recovery. CCHER is expanding its housing services within the agency to address this issue of homelessness and substance abuse.

Training of community members within the 'volunteer health educator' model must continue and the curriculum will continue to be refined. CCHER has collected pre- and post-data on the knowledge, attitudes and beliefs of Haitians from the initial groups of trainees participating in the program. This information will assist CCHER staff in planning training activities as well as for evaluating the impact of this intervention. The relative short time that the training has been taking place has limited evaluation of the model to date.

CCHER Substance Abuse Department staff find that many students enter the program with misconceptions about addiction, with a lack of understanding of how drugs and alcohol can affect the body and the brain, and how alcohol and drug use can be linked with the transmission of HIV. Because of the unfamiliarity with the American medical, social service and legal systems, many Haitians come to the training with little knowledge of the social implications of substance abuse such as the link with domestic violence, crime, and the involvement of child protection services in cases where children are involved.

There is a need for educational approaches for the illiterate as well as the literate. About three-fourths of Haiti's population is illiterate, a barrier that they bring with them to the United States. While many local Haitians in Boston continue to work hard in becoming English proficient, still a large number are unable to read or write in their native Creole. CCHER continues to work hard in planning culturally appropriate educational approaches that provide both illiterate and literate individuals with necessary health information.

Recognizing that there appears to be a high rate of deportation related to drug use among this group, appropriate interventions to curb this trend must be put into place.

CCHER staff have found that many Haitian families are unfamiliar with the process of recovery. Affected families and loved ones may not understand that the recovery process can result in a new or changed person. Confusion and misunderstanding can often occur among families once a Haitian consumer has gone through the detox process and is resuming family relations. There is a need for residential halfway homes in which both Haitian families and those in recovery can become educated about the process of recovery and be supported throughout this process.

CONCLUSION AND FUTURE DIRECTIONS

CCHER's Psychosocial Educational Counseling Curriculum (PEC), created as a result of the HRSA SPNS program, has allowed CCHER counselors to engage in in-depth counseling sessions and discussions with Haitian HIV consumers. These sessions explored the tremendous psychosocial burdens that many consumers are faced with and has brought to the forefront some important issues related to substance abuse and addiction among the Haitian community. The creation of a new Substance Abuse Department has allowed CCHER to begin collecting qualitative and quantitative information on what we think is just the tip of the iceberg of an issue that has received little attention within the Haitian community. From the existing preliminary programming strategies being put into place, CCHER is beginning to learn the needs of substance abusers in the Boston Haitian community and how best to provide culturally competent services to address those needs. Preliminary evidence suggests that if these interventions are to be effective, CCHER must develop these interventions from a community level approach. Interventions must be directed simultaneously towards consumer-centered service delivery and community action. These targeted approaches were found to be effective in addressing the HIV epidemic in the Boston Haitian community. In the future, CCHER will need to: (1) create a database of reported IDU and of the use of cocaine, crack, alcohol and other substances and their overall impact on the morbidity of the community; (2) continue to create a database of knowledge, attitudes and beliefs of the community in relation to substance abuse through culturally relevant questionnaires. Our early work has shown promise, yet there are still many limitations and challenges ahead. The primary goals of our substance abuse programming is to prevent drug use and its comorbidities and reduce the level of addiction among Haitians; more in-depth study and time will be needed to provide the necessary information about the "culture" of substance abuse and the disease of addiction among Haitians to meet these goals. More specific resources, guidance and skills will be needed so that CCHER can continue to 'unveil' this hidden problem within the community.

REFERENCES

Adrien, A., Boivin, J., Tousignant, Y., & Hankins, K. (1990). Knowledge, attitudes, beliefs and practices related to AIDS among Montreal residents of Haitian origin. *Canadian Journal of Public Health, 81*, 129-134.

Angel, R. & Guarnaccia, P. (1989). Mind, body and culture: somatization among Hispanics. *Social Science and Medicine, 28* (12), 1229-1238.

Farmer, P. (1992). *AIDS and Accusation: Haiti and the Geography of Blame.* California: University of California Press.

Fox, K., Merrill, J. C., Chang, H., & Califana, J. A. (1995). Estimating the costs of substance abuse to the Medicaid hospital care program. *American Journal of Public Health, 85*, 48-54.

Huba, G. J., Melchior, L. A., Panter, A. T., Brown, V. B., & Larson, T. A. (2000). A national program of AIDS care projects and their cross-cutting evaluation: The HRSA SPNS cooperative agreements. *Drugs & Society, 16* (1/2), 5-29.

Laguerre, M. (1981). Haitian Americans. In Harwood, A. (Ed.), *Ethnicity and Medical Care* (pp. 172-210). Cambridge: Harvard University Press.

Laguerre, M. (1984). American Odyssey: Haitians in New York City. Ithaca: Cornell University.

Leclere, F., Jensen, L., & Biddlecom, A. (1994). Health care utilization, family context, and adaptation among immigrants to the United States. *Journal of Health and Social Behavior, 35*, 370-384.

Martin, M., Rissmiller, P., & Beal, J. (1995). Health illness beliefs and practices of Haitians with HIV disease living in Boston. *Journal of the Association of Nurses in AIDS Care, 6* (6), 45-53.

Massachusetts Department of Public Health. (1998). *Refugees and Immigrants in Massachusetts: An Overview of Selected Communities.* Boston.

Massachusetts Department of Public Health. (1999, January). AIDS Surveillance Bureau Statistics.

Miller, J. (1984). *The plight of Haitian refugees.* New York: Praeger.

Preeg, E. (1996). *The Haitian dilemma: a case study in demographics, development, and U.S. foreign policy.* Washington, DC: Center for Strategic and International Studies.

Rebach, H. (1992). Alcohol and drug use among ethnic minorities. In J. Trimble,

C. Bolek, & S. Niemcryk (Eds.), *Ethnic and multicultural drug abuse: Perspectives on current research.* (pp. 23-57). New York: The Haworth Press, Inc.

Viera, J., Frank, E., Spira, T., & Landesman, S. (1983). Acquired immune deficiency in Haitians: Opportunistic infections in previously healthy Haitian immigrants. *The New England Journal of Medicine, 308* (3), 125-129.

Watson, J., Mattera, G., Morales, R., Kunitz, S., & Lynch, R. (1985). Alcohol use among migrant laborers in western New York. *Journal of Studies on Alcohol, 46,* 403-411.

Zephir, F. (1996). *Haitian immigrants in Black America: A sociological and sociolinguistical portrait.* Westport, CT: Bergin & Garvey.

The Fortune Society's Latino Discharge Planning: A Model of Comprehensive Care for HIV-Positive Ex-Offenders

Ana Motta-Moss, MA
Nicholas Freudenberg, DrPH
Wayman Young
Tracey Gallagher

SUMMARY. The Fortune Society provides outreach, discharge planning and case management for HIV-positive inmates and ex-offenders. The Latino Discharge Planning (LDP) project was designed to meet the social service needs of HIV-positive individuals who were about to be released from New York correctional facilities. This paper describes initial evaluation results of the LDP program. Most program clients are adult males (Median = 36 years of age; 89% males, 11% females), with the vast majority meeting established criteria for AIDS. The LDP model incorporates the target population's culture and transitional issues ex-

---

Ana Motta-Moss and Nicholas Freudenberg are affiliated with the Hunter College Center on AIDS, Drugs and Community Health, New York, NY. Wayman Young and Tracey Gallagher are affiliated with The Fortune Society, New York, NY.

Address correspondence to: Ana Motta-Moss, MA, Hunter College Center on AIDS, Drugs and Community Health, 425 East 25th Street #1323, New York, NY 10010 (E-mail: amoss@shiva.hunter.cuny.edu).

This work was supported in part by the Health Resources and Services Administration (HRSA), HIV/AIDS Bureau (HAB), Special Projects of National Significance (SPNS) Grant No. BRU 900107-05. This publication's contents are solely the responsibility of the authors and do not necessarily represent the official view of the funding agency.

[Haworth co-indexing entry note]: "The Fortune Society's Latino Discharge Planning: A Model of Comprehensive Care for HIV-Positive Ex-Offenders." Motta-Moss, Ana et al. Co-published simultaneously in *Drugs & Society* (The Haworth Press, Inc.) Vol. 16, No. 1/2, 2000, pp. 123-144; and: *Evaluating HIV/AIDS Treatment Programs: Innovative Methods and Findings* (ed: G. J. Huba et al.) The Haworth Press, Inc., 2000, pp. 123-144. Single or multiple copies of this article are available for a fee from The Haworth Document Delivery Service [1-800-342-9678, 9:00 a.m. - 5:00 p.m. (EST). E-mail address: getinfo@haworthpressinc.com].

offenders face in their return to society at large. Key program elements include reliance on peer services and positive role modeling, a supportive environment to encourage socially acceptable and healthier behaviors, and a holistic and advocacy-driven approach to service provision. *[Article copies available for a fee from The Haworth Document Delivery Service: 1-800-342-9678. E-mail address: <getinfo@haworthpressinc.com> Website: <http://www.HaworthPress.com>]*

KEYWORDS. Discharge planning, HIV/AIDS services, ex-offenders, intensive case management, community outreach

INTRODUCTION

A large body of research has indicated that individual-level HIV prevention interventions have been effective in changing risk-behavior in a variety of populations, such as adolescent and adult heterosexuals, gay and bisexual men, substance users, and adults with serious mental illness (Des Jarlais & Friedman, 1987; Dill, 1994; Choi & Coates, 1994; Kamb et al. 1997; Kalichman, Carey, & Johnson, 1996). In addition to HIV risk-reduction interventions, case management has been acknowledged as an important intervention model with the potential to address a variety of client needs (Rhodes & Gross, 1997; Rothman, 1991). Over time, case management intervention strategies have improved to provide greater continuity and coordination of care to persons who need a wide variety of long-term support and services (Baldwin & Woods, 1994). Little is known, however, about the implementation of HIV risk-reduction case management among populations with multiple needs, such as HIV-positive inmates and recently released ex-offenders who also struggle with substance abuse issues. This paper attempts to fulfill this gap by providing a description of an HIV risk-reduction case management model targeted specifically to HIV-positive inmates and ex-offenders.

Program Background

The Fortune Society has developed a specialized HIV case management program–Empowerment Through HIV Information, Community and Services (ETHICS)–to meet a variety of social service and treatment needs of HIV infected individuals who were about to be released or had been recently released from correctional facilities into New York City. While developing and implementing the ETHICS model, the Fortune Society became increasingly aware of the need to improve the inmates' discharge planning process. At the moment of discharge from jails and prisons, inmates often lack knowledge of available community services, making it essential that program staff conduct outreach to correctional facilities in order to ensure that needed services are available immediately upon the inmates' release.

As The Fortune Society initiated outreach activities to HIV-positive individuals in the correctional facilities, staff became increasingly aware of the special needs of this population, particularly the needs of the Latino HIV-positive inmates. Staff identified three primary characteristics of this group: (a) Latino inmates face serious problems accessing services because of the cultural and linguistic barriers unique to their varied cultures; (b) cultural beliefs reinforce the individuals' neglect of their own health-related needs, in favor of their rushing to find work and provide for the family; and (c) Latinos are over-represented in both incarceration and HIV prevalence rates. To address these concerns, The Fortune Society developed the Latino Discharge Planning Project.

Project Orientation, Strategies and Objectives

The LDP is a comprehensive model program that has been developed to reach out to the increasing population of HIV-positive Latino inmates and ex-offenders. The program targets individuals who are in the process of making a transition from the New York State prisons and New York City jails into community life. The overall goals of the LDP program are: (a) to provide a humane transition to the community for inmates who are HIV-positive and symptomatic, and (b) to ensure that the clients' basic needs–medical, drug treatment, social support, educational/vocational, nutritional, housing, and legal–will be met upon their release from the correctional facilities.

The program model includes seven components:

- Identification and initial contact with potential program participants;
- Administration of initial intake protocols with eligible inmates;
- Development of a discharge plan addressing health and social service needs upon release;
- On-going client contact prior to release;
- Social integration of newly-released LDP clients with active ETHICS clients;
- Provision of intensive counseling, case management and support services for clients; and
- Provision of referrals and follow-up contacts for additional services at other organizations.

METHOD

Subjects

Originally, the LDP project exclusively targeted HIV-positive symptomatic Latino inmates and parolees. Because of the pragmatic difficulties and ethical implications of refusing services to individuals of other ethnic groups or to those who are HIV-positive but still asymptomatic, The Fortune Society has redefined this objective to include a broader target population. Currently, while the LDP project maintains its focus on Latino clients, it also enrolls approximately 25% of clients who come from other ethnic backgrounds and/or are not yet HIV symptomatic.

The LDP project goal is to provide discharge planning to approximately 175 inmates at New York City and New York State correctional facilities every year. In addition, the program is designed to engage 75 of these inmates in the community-based portion of the program upon their release from jail/prison. Although the LDP project still aims to achieve these objectives, greater emphasis has been placed on refining the recruitment, engagement, and retention strategies, and the organizational structure of the LDP model of service delivery in order to most efficiently and effectively address the overall goals of the project. The local evaluation, in turn, has focused on these efforts.

Design and Procedure

With the objective of describing and examining the implementation of the LDP project, evaluation staff from Hunter College Center on AIDS, Drugs and Community Health utilized a combination of qualitative and quantitative analytic techniques. The methods used to document and evaluate the implementation phase of the LDP project include:

Staff interviews. Semi-structured face-to-face interviews were conducted with the six (6) line staff and managers directly involved in the LDP project. The objectives of these interviews were to: (a) clarify the information about the strategies used and barriers faced during recruitment, engagement, and retention of clients in the program; (b) describe referral and follow-up procedures; (c) identify existing supervisory and support mechanisms for staff; and (d) elicit suggestions for improving the implementation of the project.

Client chart reviews. In an effort to examine the characteristics of the LDP client population and the patterns of service provision, evaluation staff selected a stratified sample of 46 client charts for review. The selection of the charts was based on the client status in the program: (a) incarcerated clients who were initially contacted in jail/prison between October and January, 1995, but were not enrolled as community-based clients as of April 8, 1996 (LDP/1), and (b) parolees who were enrolled and actively receiving services in the community-based LDP program at Fortune as of April 8, 1996 (LDP/2). These two sets of clients (n = 34 LDP/1; n = 12 LDP/2) were selected in order to secure information on a diverse and representative range of clients who were recruited and/or actively enrolled in the LDP program during the federal fiscal year 1996. The data extracted from the client charts include: (1) socio-demographic characteristics, (2) date and type of initial contact, admission in and discharge from the program, (3) LDP program status (as described above) and correctional facility in which client was contacted, (4) number of staff/client contacts per month during incarceration, (5) HIV status and year of diagnosis, drug history and frequency of usage, (6) identified client needs, service referrals and follow-up procedures, and (7) services provided, including number of case management sessions (in person and by telephone), support groups, escort to services, hospital visits, and home visits.

RESULTS

Project data collected through May 31, 1996, are described below to present some key features in the service model as implemented.

Staff Characteristics

As of May 1996, the LDP project of The Fortune Society was fully staffed with six (6) full-time staff, including an administrative assistant, two.case manager/outreach workers, a project outreach coordinator, a project director, and a senior counselor. Although agency staff have worked at The Fortune Society for an average of one and a half years, most of the LDP staff are fairly new to the project. Two (33%) staff have been with LDP for six months or less, three (50%) have been involved in the program for 6-12 months, and only one (17%) staff member, the Project Director, has been with the LDP since the program's onset two years earlier.

While the LDP staff do not entirely match clients in terms of ethnic background, they do meet the linguistic needs of the Latino community they serve in that three of the LDP direct line staff speak Spanish fluently. In terms of gender, the staff are evenly distributed between males ($n = 3$) and females ($n = 3$). In addition, the age range of the staff, 30-45 years old, coincide with that of the project's target population. Most staff share with the LDP clients either a history of prior incarceration or an HIV-positive status, factors that they feel are essential to providing discharge planning services to HIV-positive ex-offenders. In the view of staff members, however, *"it is not easy to find the right person, within or outside the community, with the appropriate skills, understanding, and commitment to work with HIV-positive ex-offenders."*

Overall, the LDP staff expressed a high level of motivation to perform their tasks and a strong commitment to their clients. Their motivation and commitment are based on factors such as an AIDS-related death in their own families, prior contact with other Fortune staff during their own incarceration experience, prior experience as an HIV/AIDS counselor/health educator, and the support and training received from other Fortune staff while on work release.

While not atypical during the early stages of a new and demanding program, the LDP experienced a high turnover during its first two years of operation.[1] Although no data on the consequences of the high turnover rate are available, it is likely to have affected the program's efforts to establish on-going relationships with the LDP clients as well as to maintaining relationships with correctional facilities' staff and parole officers. Nonetheless, contacts with other community-based organizations, especially those serving HIV-positive individuals and their families, have been maintained by the Fortune staff responsible for the dissemination of the program model. In addition, access to new upstate facilities has been secured through the efforts of agency managers.

Staff Supervision, Support Mechanisms, and Training

Several mechanisms, formal and informal, are used to supervise and monitor the work performed by the LDP staff. These mechanisms include folder review, weekly supervision, case conference, and weekly unit meetings.

The case management portion of the program is submitted to a quality control process that involves folder reviews once weekly. Assigned managers and staff review client charts and check for the frequency and accuracy of the documentation in the charts. This process allows reviewers to identify problems in service provision as well as documentation, and address them with the staff. For instance, during one of the LDP staff meetings, the issue of verification of referrals was brought up as one that needed clarification to ensure consistency: some staff were verifying a referral as "accepted" after they had confirmed that clients had gone to the referral agency while other staff would check that category only after the client had been accepted into the program to which he/she was referred.

Two-hour group supervision sessions are also scheduled on a weekly basis among the senior coordinators and case managers/counselors. These sessions focus primarily on administrative issues involving agency policies and procedures, although they can also be used for updates and exchange of resources (e.g., about referral sites). In addition, the LDP staff rely on the assistance of a consultant who facilitates monthly clinical case conferences in which selected client cases are discussed. The LDP staff believe the case conferences offer an opportunity to have in-house practical training based on their own work.

With regard to clinical and administrative training, staff pointed out that because they are required to help clients who have multiple needs, their training demands are extended beyond what is usually provided at Fortune. As expressed by a staff member, "*one needs to be multi-tasked and multi-faceted in terms of talent in order to work on the LDP program.*" The LDP staff provide outreach, case management and counseling, crisis intervention, discharge planning, and referrals. At times, they feel that it is difficult to manage the demands of these different roles. To prepare staff for this multitude of roles, Fortune offers internal training that focuses primarily on case management-required documentation and procedures, and group presentation skills. Training on other content areas, such as supervisory skills, counseling, and HIV-related clinical trials are offered to staff at outside agencies.

Population Served

Consistent with the focus of the LDP project, approximately three-quarters of the combined sample of clients reached during the fiscal year were Latinos (74%), and a little less than 20% were African Americans (see Table 1 for specific clients' sociodemographic information). With regard to HIV status, two-thirds of the clients were HIV-positive and symptomatic (67%), with the vast majority of these fulfilling the criteria for CDC-defined AIDS (52%), and one-third (33%) were HIV-infected and not yet symptomatic. Typically, LDP clients have been diagnosed with HIV within the past five years. Age and gender distributions of the sample indicate that the population served by the LDP project is comprised predominantly of males in their 30s (Median = 36 years of age; 89% males, 11% females). More than three-quarters (80%) of the community clients had a history of prior substance use, and approximately one-third were in recovery and required additional services to sustain their efforts. In addition, 36% of the clients had secured public assistance upon release, primarily through the efforts of the advocacy work of the LDP staff. Still, over 50% of the clients had no means of support upon release.

The following strategies have been utilized by Fortune staff to facilitate the recruitment of clients for the LDP program as well as provide discharge planning.

Visits to the correctional facilities. Every third week of each month, two Fortune staff–an outreach worker and a case manager–conduct visits to correctional facilities in upstate New York. During these visits, staff perform group presentations on the services provided at Fortune, and also address HIV prevention and healthcare and discuss relevant entitlement programs. In addition, staff talk with inmates individually about their specific service needs. Also during these visits, the staff may hold meetings with correctional facilities' administrative and pre-release office staff, with the objective of dealing with issues related to the clearance of program staff. In New York City, staff conduct outreach visits at Rikers Correctional Facility twice every month.

In all facilities, the LDP staff conduct a brief eligibility assessment during individual interviews with inmates. If the inmate's characteristics and needs fit the LDP selection criterion (Latino HIV-positive inmates to be released from prison within six months),[2] the staff continue with the discharge planning process. The discharge plan includes identification of client needs upon

TABLE 1. Sociodemographic Characteristics of Clients by LDP Program Status

Number of Clients per Program Status	LDP/1 n = 34 (100%) (Still in jail/prison)	LDP/2 n = 12 (100%) (Active community clients)	TOTAL n = 46 (100%)
Gender			
Male	29 (85)	12 (100)	41 (89)
Female	5 (15)	--	5 (11)
Ethnicity			
Latino/a	24 (71)	10 (83)	34 (74)
African American	8 (23)	--	8 (17)
White	1 (3)	2 (17)	3 (7)
Native American	1 (3)	--	1 (2)
Education			
Less than High School	11 (50)	5 (42)	16 (47)
High School/GED	8 (36)	6 (50)	14 (41)
More than High School	3 (14)	1 (8)	4 (12)
Missing	12	--	12
Income			
Public Assistance	N/A	7 (64)	7 (64)
Family &/or spouse	N/A	--	--
None	N/A	4 (36)	4 (36)
Other	N/A	--	--
Missing	N/A	1	1
Age*	35 (29-54)	39 (31-57)	36 (29-57)
Years since HIV Diagnosis*	5 (1-14)	7 (1-11)	5 (1-14)

*Medium Range

release and gathering necessary documentation (e.g., birth certificates, social security card) that will allow inmates to access needed health and social services upon their release from prison. Upon release, these clients are enrolled in case management, counseling, and other services at The Fortune Society. Those inmates who do not meet the selection criterion for participation in the LDP program are referred to other organizations for services after their release from prison.

Information from the chart reviews indicates that clients were reached at 22 facilities located in New York City, the larger New York City Region, and

Upstate New York.[3] The majority of the clients were reached in Upstate New York facilities (n = 30; 67%), followed by Rikers Island in New York City (n = 11, 24%) and other correctional facilities in the New York City Region (n = 4, 9%). Overall, the LDP staff believe that visiting the correctional facilities is one of the most powerful forms of outreach. As stated by a staff member,

> *Although there is not enough time to do everything during the visits (identification of clients, group presentation, individual interviews, contact facilities' personnel, etc.), face-to-face contacts with inmates is the most powerful strategy for reaching clients because it may be the inmates' only contact with the outside world. It facilitates identification between staff and clients because of the staff personal background experiences in prison her/himself–it lets them know that there is life after prison–it builds immediate trust because of the similarities between staff and inmates.*

Nonetheless, the outreach visits to upstate facilities can be a burdensome strategy. It requires a broad range of preparatory work in order to obtain.staff clearance and it involves about six hours traveling from New York City to upstate prisons. Because it takes so long for the staff to travel to and from the facilities, they need to stay overnight, which takes their time away from being with their families. Moreover, the clearance process in practically all state facilities involves scheduling their visits, specifying day, hour, and length of time the staff are going to be there, and in some facilities, the presence of an escort to guide and monitor staff into the facility. In addition, occasional incidents or disciplinary actions in the facilities result in a "lock down," rendering the trip useless because the staff are denied access to the inmates.

Mailing campaigns. Mailing campaigns are conducted through the network of social service organizations that work inside the correctional facilities. Staff from those organizations distribute LDP flyers/information to the inmates they have contact with, providing the inmates with the information on how to access services at Fortune. They also contact Fortune staff on behalf of the inmates whom they know need those services. The initial contact between the LDP staff and potential clients may occur either in person or by mail or telephone, and follow-up contact is kept on a monthly basis. This strategy is mostly used with the facilities that are located outside of the New York City region, with a particular focus on those facilities at which Fortune staff do not have clearance to access. As a manager stated, *"This strategy works well. It is set up as a safety net to facilitate access to the LDP program."*

Some of the challenges faced by staff in using the mailing campaigns to recruit clients for the LDP program include the literacy level of clients, movement of inmates within the same facility or to other facilities (without notice to LDP staff), changes in inmates' status due to disciplinary actions within the facility, and illness of clients (i.e., they are too sick to write). In addition, mailing campaigns require more initiative from inmates in trying to establish and maintain the contact with program staff. A program manager believes that one of the limitations of mailing as a recruitment strategy is that even if 50 clients were reached by mailing, Fortune does not have the staff power to keep in contact with those 50 people on a monthly basis for six months, and effectively track them down through the changes while getting things ready for their release. Thus, outreach visits are also utilized to maintain contact with inmates during the discharge planning process.

Secondary linkages. The LDP staff also utilize the relationships that have been previously established with criminal justice personnel, community agencies, and inmates to foster the recruitment of clients to the program. Recruitment strategies used through these community linkages include: (a) meetings with parole officers to identify potential clients and promote referrals to services at Fortune; (b) regular contact with staff from other community-based organizations that provide services within correctional facilities and/or to ex-offenders; and (c) identification of informal Latino inmate groups within the correctional facilities.

Overall information from the chart reviews indicates that more than half (57%, $n = 26$) of the LDP clients were initially contacted during the staff visits to correctional facilities, with 30% ($n = 14$) of the clients being contacted through letters, and 6% ($n = 13$) through the telephone.

Analysis of the information on the length of time between initial contact and admission in the LDP program at The Fortune Society is consistent with the program objective of reaching inmates who are within six months of their release from prison/jail. Overall, the median length of time between the initial contact in jail/prison and the admission into the program is of about four (4) months, with a median number of staff/client contacts of about one-and-a-half contacts per month. According to the staff, sometimes, even when inmates have their parole board meetings and are denied release from prison, Fortune staff will still keep in contact with them, and *"let them know that they have not been forgotten."*

Engagement Strategies

The transition back into the community can be and typically is traumatic for LDP clients. After learning to manage their lives within the prison or jail system, clients must learn anew how to meet their needs, particularly their immediate medical, financial, and housing needs. To every extent possible, LDP staff try to meet clients released from upstate facilities at the New York ⌐ity bus station. The staff establish a supportive relationship while accompanying the client to the Fortune facility. Similarly, the staff ensure that clients released from Rikers Island (city jail) have an appointment scheduled at

Fortune on the same day of their release. Once at The Fortune Society, the staff work with the client to identify and address his/her immediate needs. In interviews, staff identified the two most common kinds of "offerings" they typically make to the client: they help the client identify an immediate place to stay and they provide clients with food and clothes. The staff also make available to clients a "community voice mail." This service provides an anonymous and convenient way for the clients to communicate with staff and other individuals, and it is particularly useful if clients have not disclosed their HIV status to family members. The service can also be very helpful in job searches and for those clients who do not have easy access to a telephone. These offerings not only address the clients' needs but they help to bond the clients to the LDP program and its staff.

A key aspect of the engagement process comprises assisting clients in securing the support of their families. In such cases, and always with the clients' permission, the staff work jointly with the clients and their families. According to the staff, the LDP clients and their family members often need help in talking about and addressing the client's HIV status and the HIV status of family members. They need help in talking about treatment options and about re-infection. The LDP staff believe that by strengthening the bond and support between clients and their families, they will facilitate the integration of clients back to the community and further engage clients in the program.

LDP staff also strive to secure the support of their clients' parole officers. Usually, clients are required to contact their parole officers within 24 hours of their release during which time the LDP staff describe the kinds of services they offer to the parole officers. Agency staff often point out that it is in the officers' best interest to support their parolees in services at The Fortune Society. As one staff member stated: "*if the clients are engaged in health and social services, they are less likely to get in trouble.*" Clients, in turn, do not want to alienate their parole officers.

In addition to client characteristics and program engagement strategies, events during the incarceration period can affect the client engagement in the community portion of the program. As indicated earlier, some clients are moved without notice to the LDP staff from one facility to another, while other clients have their prison status or release date changed because of a disciplinary action.

Retention Strategies

According to the LDP staff, the strategies used to retain clients in the community-based program include: (a) making sure clients receive all entitlement and benefits he/she applies for (note that 50% of the clients have no source of support upon release), (b) working on issues of substance abuse treatment, permanent housing, and medical care, (c) facilitating a bond among clients, staff, and other ex-offenders, (d) offering an accepting atmosphere at the agency, and (e) assisting clients in their negotiations with parole officers, including *"eliciting support for treatment by encouraging clients to disclose their HIV status to their officers,"* and *"encouraging clients to keep their relationship with parole officers in good standards,"* through keeping scheduled visits and contacts in order to increase the officers' trust in the clients' rehabilitation.

One of the main objectives of the LDP program is to create an atmosphere of support for its clients. As stated by one staff, *"at Fortune, you don't need to hide your identity as an ex-criminal anymore."* Client support groups, for instance, are built around thematic areas (e.g., substance use, family, sexual assault, discrimination), yet the common theme is that everybody is an ex-offender. In addition, case managers assist clients in dealing with their criminal justice issues (e.g., court appeals, representation in court). As said by a staff member, *"there is compassion in handling the clients' cases. We advocate for our clients."*

Findings[4] from the information gathered in the chart reviews suggest that clients who are recruited from New York upstate facilities tend to stay engaged in the community-based program longer than those clients recruited in the city. In addition, preliminary analyses suggest that the longer Fortune staff work with clients while s/he is incarcerated, the more likely it is that the client will stay in the community-based LDP program for a longer period of time.

The Fortune Society has an open-door policy which means that the *"clients know they can always come back."* The LDP staff also provide activities, such as movie tickets, computer laboratory training for the development of marketable job skills, and tokens for clients to come to Fortune for services.

Barriers to client retention. As described by Fortune managers, the LDP staff often try to help clients who do not necessarily fall into the selection criteria for the LDP program (for instance, inmates from a different ethnic background, HIV-positive asymptomatic Latino ex-offenders, and families of the LDP clients). While this approach is in accordance with the mission of The Fortune Society, the provision of these services relies on available staff resources, diminishing their ability to further develop retention strategies. In attempting to describe how this situation adds yet another layer on the stack of staff responsibilities, a staff stated that,

> *One of the barriers [to client services] is that some clients do not fit under any of the new categories of funding at Fortune, which implies that our resources are stretched to the limit of our capacity. We deliver needed services through whatever resources we have, and then provide necessary referrals.*

One of the barriers to client retention mentioned by staff resides in the reluctance by some clients to discuss issues related to their illness (AIDS or substance abuse-related issues). As a staff member pointed out, *"some clients show a lack of interest about or feel uncomfortable in participating in on-going programs to discuss issues they may not yet be ready to talk about."*

Another factor identified by staff as a barrier to client retention in the program refers to the limited variety of mechanisms for client involvement and participation. Staff believe that for some clients, *"once their basic needs (housing, entitlement, and healthcare) are met they do not want to stay to participate in the support groups or on-going case management/counseling."* Most LDP staff believe that additional components such as speakers' bureau and buddy programs would be helpful. About half of the client charts reviewed provide information about clients who are still engaged in the LDP program. Data from the 21 clients already discharged, however, indicate that most clients were lost to contact (*n* = 8, 38%) or exited the program by their own initiative (*n* = 6, 27%). Of the remaining clients, three (14%) were referred by staff to another program, two (10.5%) were deceased, and two (10.5%) were re-arrested.

Most staff believe that the desired outcome of the LDP project is to assist HIV-positive ex-offenders in their reintegration back to the community. They also think that their main mission is to meet the clients' immediate needs–healthcare, housing, entitlements–in order to provide a certain degree of stabilization to their lives. According to this view, the needs of the LDP clients go far beyond medical, housing or entitlement issues: clients need hope, support, and opportunity to rebuild their lives upon release from prison.

Referral Strategies

After the initial assessment of the needs of potential clients, outreach staff may provide inmates with a referral for services at The Fortune Society or at outside organizations. In general, those clients who are not coming to New York City upon release and those who require services not provided at Fortune (e.g., residential drug treatment programs) are referred to needed services at organizations in their area of release.

Those inmates who come into New York City upon release are engaged in the LDP community-based services at Fortune. Depending on Fortune's ability to meet some or all of the clients' needs, certain services are provided by the LDP staff (e.g., case management/counseling, support group meetings, HIV/AIDS education, legal assistance, job training) while others are provided at outside agencies (e.g., healthcare, entitlement, housing). One of the LDP staff describes the referral process as follows:

> *When a client tells me 'all I need is a healthcare provider. I don't want to go to no group and I don't want one-on-one counseling . . . I am alright, just get me hooked up with a doctor,' I then refer him/her to a hospital nearest to them. We go with them to make an appointment. We*

> *give them the name, date of birth, current T-cell count, and any medical records we have–they are faxed to them at the hospital. Then, we get the client an appointment, and that's it. Unless the client wants to come back here. We always let them know that this is home. I tell all my guys that: 'This is home. Whenever you feel shaky, come here. This is safe.'*

Some of the barriers to referrals identified by the LDP staff refer to the fact that other agencies may have expertise in HIV care but not in criminal justice issues. These barriers include resistance from staff of other social service agencies to accept clients who are ex-offenders, lack of experience and skills of case managers in those agencies to help clients with their criminal justice issues (e.g., negotiations with parole officers), and the clients' belief that they need to hide their history of incarceration from staff at those agencies in order to receive appropriate services. Usually, the LDP staff call the staff at outside agencies as a means to follow-up on the referrals provided to clients. In addition, staff discuss with clients whether or not they are satisfied with the services received at the outside agencies.

According to the LDP staff, two factors facilitate the referral of clients to outside agencies: (1) the formal and informal linkages established between The Fortune Society and several health and social service agencies, and (2) the personal resources and skills of the LDP staff. The most common scenario is that of an LDP staff contacting someone they know at another agency and checking about the immediate availability of needed services for their clients. Sometimes, staff from other agencies call their LDP contact and let he/she know about the availability of specific services (e.g., housing). The following description by a staff member illustrates their caring and committed attitude to the referral of clients to other agencies:

> *We have linkages with several agencies in New York City. Sometimes, their staff reach out to us and say: 'listen, we have this bed space to give you.' What happens is that we have to go out and check it out and see what the conditions are. Our hearts are on it, before we send any of our guys out, we say: 'would I?'*

Client Service Needs

The combined information from staff reports and chart reviews indicate that the most frequently identified needs among the LDP community-based clients refer to medical care ($n = 32$, 97%), case management/counseling ($n = 30$, 91%), and legal services ($n = 25$, 76%). These primary client needs required the provision of healthcare, entitlement for public assistance/social benefits, and housing services. Specific frequencies of needs and referrals provided are presented in Table 2.

In addition to the previously identified needs, staff believe that secondary

TABLE 2. Identified Client Needs and Frequency of Referrals by Areas of Need (N = 33)

Identified Needs and Referrals	Total Number of Charts Reviewed N (%)
Medical	
Need*	32 (97)
Referral**	29 (91)
Psychological	
Need*	21 (64)
Referral**	19 (90)
Counseling	
Need*	30 (91)
Referral**	26 (87)
Social	
Need*	24 (73)
Referral**	22 (92)
Vocational	
Need*	5 (15)
Referral**	2 (40)
Nutritional	
Need*	24 (73)
Referral**	13 (54)
Legal	
Need*	25 (76)
Referral**	24 (96)

*Frequency of community clients presenting specific need.
**Out of those clients with specific needs, frequency of referrals.

needs of clients include social support, legal advocacy, HIV/AIDS prevention/treatment education, recovery readiness and support, and community acceptance and reintegration. The process of providing these services is complex and requires a strong commitment from staff.

In general, clients expect that The Fortune Society, as an agency, will assist them in obtaining the social, health, substance use, educational, and legal services they need. As stated by a staff member, *"clients are looking for assistance because many of them are afraid to speak for themselves or do not know about their rights."* From the LDP program, *"clients want support, a safe haven . . . a place where they are welcome at any time.*" From the staff, clients expect more than just professionals who provide services,

> *I know they want a friend, someone they can tell anything to, and know that [whatever they say] is not going to pass this door . . . unless it is something like . . . committing suicide. I have a 56 year old [client] with me that calls me 'Ma.' [He says] 'I do whatever you tell me, Ma.' It's kind of strange . . . Even when I go out to the prison they [inmates] have coffee, cake, sandwiches [for me] . . . They are waiting out for me, in their wheelchairs, they are coming out the gate . . . [They say] 'Me first Ma.' I go to each one of their beds, hold them . . . they hold my hand. I let them know that there is someone out there [for them]. A lot of them have no family, or they have done so much damage that they burn their bridges and the families don't care anymore. I don't promise anything, [but] I fight tooth and nail and they see me arguing with doctors out there . . . I had to be escorted out of the Island once because I blew up at a doctor. She [the doctor] would not write up a medical report that I needed to get this man into a nursing home.*

Typically, clients come to Fortune twice a week for a variety of services, including counseling, support groups, computer classes, and job training. Most of the staff think that clients should come to Fortune more often, "*to prevent them from getting into trouble.*" Preliminary analyses of the information provided on clients who have been discharged from the program suggest that the median length of client stay in the program is about two and a half months (Median = 2.4, Range: 1-6 months). Although the length of stay in the program may vary according to the clients' needs, staff try to keep them engaged as long as possible, "*until their transition back to the community becomes more stable.*"

Secondary analyses of the information from chart reviews[5] indicate that those clients who were involved in the program after October 1, 1995 had more face-to-face case management/counseling sessions per month ($M = 5.0$, $SD = 4.03$) than those contacted prior to that date ($M = 2.9$, $SD = 3.05$). No significant differences were found in the number of telephone/mail contact or attendance in support group sessions among these two groups.

As perceived by staff, case management and counseling services for HIV-positive symptomatic ex-offenders require special considerations. A staff member stated, "*LDP counseling is about coping skills, patience, spirituality, restoring hope in the clients' lives.*" Often, beyond the issues of illness and death, staff are the only people with whom clients can discuss their anger, fear, sadness, frustration, and/or plans. The following paragraph illustrates the trust that exists between staff and the LDP clients:

> *Clients usually feel safe with me. They come here and tell me: 'Look at this' . . . One day a guy came in here and handed me a box cutter and said: 'I'm going to kill her [his girlfriend] . . . I brought this to you because I'm going to kill her . . . Take this before I end up in jail for the rest of my life.'*

Although staff think that the LDP program meets most of the needs of its target population, they feel that the clients' issues with substance abuse still require additional resources in order to be adequately addressed in the program. While a few of the staff favor harm-reduction in dealing with the clients' substance abuse issues, they perceive that the organizational capacity at The Fortune Society favors a risk-reduction approach, which is not always effective for those clients who are not ready to change their drug-using behaviors.

Lessons Learned

During the first two years of program implementation, The Fortune Society fulfilled the overall goals of the LDP program: establishing and operating an innovative program that assists HIV infected Latino and other inmates in their return back to neighborhood life in New York City. The LDP staff have consistently provided case management services to help clients secure needed community-based services as well as assisted inmates in obtaining needed documents that make them eligible for these services upon their release from city jails or state prisons. Indeed, information from client chart reviews reinforces the need for such a program, illustrated most dramatically by the findings that fifty percent of the LDP clients have no source of income upon release (still others secured public assistance through the early intervention of the LDP staff) and by the fact that nearly all LDP clients indicated a need for assistance in securing medical care (which is particularly critical given their HIV status).

The LDP program has developed appropriate strategies to recruit clients throughout the New York State prison system and from Rikers Island and has secured access to 22 separate prisons and jails. Furthermore, the LDP staff have reached the target population for which the program was designed. Three-quarters of the recruited inmates are Latino and all are HIV-positive. The staff has also been successful in targeting clients who are released within six months of initial program contact: the median length of time between initial contact in jail or prison and the admission into the community-based portion of the program averages four months.

The program has also developed strategies to engage and retain clients in the program. Knowing how difficult the transition back to the community can be for their clients, LDP staff attempt to meet clients at the City bus station on their return home or to instruct clients incarcerated in City jails to meet them directly at The Fortune Society headquarters. The staff initiate the process of securing the trust of their clients by helping them meet their most immediate needs such as temporary housing, medical care, food, and clothing. In order to retain clients in the program the staff inform clients of the entitlements for which they are eligible and advocate for and with their clients to secure their entitlements. The LDP staff also help their clients maintain a good working relationship with their parole officers and the staff also attempts to integrate their clients into the client social support network in place at Fortune. The culturally syntonic environment at Fortune also provides an enticement for clients to remain active in the program.

Despite the progress The Fortune Society has made in implementing the LDP program, data from staff interviews and client chart reviews revealed several challenges that the agency has faced in the implementation of the LDP program model. These challenges are described below along with corresponding plans for addressing each of them.

Staffing and Administration

The combination of fieldwork (e.g., outreach to correctional facilities) and case management/counseling has been burdensome and unduly stressful to staff, and perceived by them as an inefficient use of their time. Alternative staff deployment strategies have been discussed. The most logical approach–as perceived by LDP staff and the evaluation team–is to have a single staff member exclusively conduct all prison/jail outreach activities. In addition, in-person outreach can be limited to those facilities that have produced the highest number of LDP clients. Letter and telephone campaigns can be used to recruit clients at the remaining facilities, particularly those where networked agencies can assist in identifying clients.

Like HIV caregivers in other settings, the LDP staff have routinely addressed their clients' fears, rage, and denial about their disease; the debilitating effects of AIDS; and in some instances the death of their clients. This work has been emotionally draining and the LDP staff expressed a need for emotional support. Increased access to supportive services for staff (e.g., support groups) addressing the emotional concerns of HIV caretakers, as well as individual counseling, has been made easily accessible to all LDP staff. A list of consultants and available staff support resources has been suggested to Fortune administrators and distributed among staff.

While not a focus of this article, it is apparent from the number of clients recruited and engaged during the second year of operations that the LDP objectives of recruiting 175 incarcerated clients and engaging 75 of those clients in the community portion of the program were met with difficulty. Because of the complexity and range of activities and services provided by the LDP program, these objectives seem unrealistically high. Considering the LDP intervention model–HIV risk-reduction intensive case management and social services–and the program's direct line staffing pattern, the yearly objective of recruiting 175 HIV-positive Latino inmates and engaging 75 of these clients into the community-based portion of the program needed to be revised.

Program Services

Due to the demands of program implementation during the first two years, the LDP staff have had reduced opportunities to facilitate the active participation and involvement of clients in program activities that did not directly involve services. Structured mechanisms for client involvement and participation in the LDP project have been devised to take place in several forms. LDP clients may provide and receive peer-led training on selected and requested topics, e.g., safer sex practices. The clients' peer educators (who are knowledgeable about a specific topic or could be referred for training-for-trainers) may be selected by staff according to a specific set of criteria. These criteria could include: client engagement in the LDP community-based program; recommendation letter from his/her counselor; and prior experience in or expertise about HIV-related issues. In addition, clients may escort other clients to needed services, select and arrange field trips or recreational activities, and secure outside speakers for workshops.

Formal mechanisms to establish social and support networks among LDP clients and other Fortune clients could facilitate exchange of resources among clients as well as peer support for reintegration into the community and substance abuse recovery. Several mechanisms to establish social and support networks among LDP clients and other Fortune clients have been considered. Some would evolve from the mechanisms described above. A client buddy system and a client-led empowerment group are other suggested formats.

Throughout the first two years of program implementation, there have been no clearly established policies or criteria to assess client success in the LDP program. Some LDP staff believed that meeting the clients' immediate needs constitutes success and some believed that client success is reflected in the clients' stable reintegration back into the community. While neither of these views is couched in time frames, the former suggests a shorter period of retention in the program than the latter. The literature on HIV care suggests that intensive case management and aftercare should be provided for a minimum of six months. The LDP staff and Fortune administrators, in consultation with the funders, have initiated discussions about establishing feasible and specific criteria for client success in the program. The implications of such criteria with regard to staffing patterns and caseload size must be carefully considered. One arrangement that could limit the LDP caseload size would involve procedures for effectively transferring clients to a less intensive case management service, either through other Fortune programs or through other agencies.

Data, Documentation and Information System

Despite having a relatively sound computerized data entry structure, data from the LDP program have not been regularly or consistently entered in the information system. This inconsistency short-circuits a potentially valuable means through which almost immediate feedback about the program could be secured. It also meant that the evaluation team had to extract data from individual client charts instead of from computerized files. Technical assistance on program documentation is recommended to implement a more consistent, coordinated, efficient, and effective way to handle the information from the LDP project. These data handling systems and procedures need to be integrated into the agency-wide information system by the IS department to ensure internal quality control. Once these improvements are implemented, a method of regularly and routinely summarizing pertinent data should be established in order to provide feedback to staff and administrators on program operations. For example, the number of clients expected to be released into the program and the number of clients who are scheduled for termination during each upcoming month could be tracked to ensure appropriate caseload sizes. In addition, the LDP client intake and assessment forms do not clearly demarcate client needs; e.g., case management and counseling needs are grouped together even though virtually all clients receive case management services and clients' emotional needs are typically addressed through case management as one of several needs. Similarly, housing needs are grouped under "legal" needs despite reflecting a very separate and important need and service. A review of client intake and assessment forms has been identified as essential to clearly demarcate client needs, particularly as they entail directly to HIV-related care.

Despite the limitations in the data available to evaluate the LDP program, this article presents valuable information about the implementation of the HIV integrated care model developed by The Fortune Society. The value and benefit of this evaluation should be considered within a context where community-based organizations, especially in ethnic minority communities, are in the process of building an infrastructure that will enable them to meet the program evaluation demands of the second decade of the AIDS epidemic. Many community-based organizations, including The Fortune Society, have limited resources to undergo evaluations, and often perceive outcome evaluation requirements as overwhelming and extremely onerous to existing programmatic and personnel resources. In order to develop the organizational conditions and commitment required by these evaluations, community-based organizations seem to require extensive technical assistance and support.

In general, the findings presented here suggest that while an outcome evaluation will ultimately be required and informative, it would be premature to begin developing strategies to conduct such an evaluation before addressing the programmatic and organizational issues discussed earlier. At the early stages of program development and implementation, community-based organizations should be focused on refining program goals, demonstrating their ability to reach target populations, monitoring the implementation of program strategies (e.g., case management, counseling, support and education), and appropriately documenting the delivery of services. As the programs develop and these initial issues are effectively addressed, community-based organizations will be better prepared for achieving more complex outcome evaluation goals.

NOTES

1. Precise data on turnover rate were not available to the evaluation team.

2. As indicated earlier, the program targets Latino inmates but does not limit enrollment exclusively to members of that ethnic group.

3. NY City: (Rikers Island)
   NY Region (Less than one and a half hour car ride from the City)
   Upstate (all other facilities)

4. Pearson = 4.53, $p < .10$; ($t_{(17)} = -2.34, p < .05$, respectively.

Note. These findings are based on a statistical comparison between clients who stayed in the program *three or more months* and those who were terminated from the program in *less than three months.*

5. $t_{(25)} = -2.18, p < .05$

Note. These findings are based on a statistical comparison between clients who stayed in the program *three or more months* and those who were terminated from the program in *less than three months.*

REFERENCES

Baldwin, S. and Woods, P. A. (1994). Case management and needs assessment: Some issues of concern for the caring professions. *Journal of Mental Health, 3,* 311-322.

Choi, K. H. and Coates, T. J. (1994). Prevention of HIV infection. *AIDS, 8,* 1371-1389.

Des Jarlais, D. C. and Friedman, S. R. (1987). HIV infection among intravenous drug users: Epidemiology and risk reduction. *AIDS, 1,* 67-76.

Dill, A. (1994). Institutional environments and organizational responses to AIDS. *Journal of Health and Social Behavior, 35,* 349-369.

Kalichman, S. C., Carey, M. P., & Johnson, B. P. (1996). Prevention of sexually transmitted HIV infection: A meta-analytic review of the behavioral outcome literature. *Annals of Behavioral Medicine, 18,* 6-15.

Kamb, M., Rhodes, F., Bolan, G., Zenilman, J., Douglas, J. M., Iatesta, M. Graziano, S., Peterman, T. & Fisherbein, M. (1997). *Does STD/HIV prevention counseling work? Preliminary results from a multi-center randomized controlled trial (Proj-*

ect Respect). Presented at the 4th Conference on Retrovirus and Opportunistic Infections, Washington, DC.

Rhodes, W. and Gross, M. (1997). *Case management reduces drug use and criminality among drug-involved arrestees: An experimental study of an HIV prevention intervention*. Report presented to the National Institute of Justice and the National Institute on Drug Abuse.

Rothman, J. (1991). A model of case management: Toward empirically-based practice. *Social Work, 36*, 520-528.

The Impact of an Intervention Program for HIV-Positive Women on Well-Being, Substance Use, Physical Symptoms, and Depression

Elaine M. Hockman, PhD
Marcia Andersen, PhD, RN, FAAN, CS
Geoffrey A. D. Smereck, AB, JD

SUMMARY. The Women's Intervention Program of the Well-Being Institute (WBI) in Detroit, Michigan, was designed to assist HIV-positive women with a history of substance abuse to access primary medical care. The program, based on The Personalized Nursing LIGHT Model, postulates that improved well-being precedes positive change in important areas such as substance use and coping with chronic disease. This evaluative study of 55 participants from intake to first follow-up after six months in the program shows that well-being significantly improved, that substance use declined as well-being improved, that well-being was a significant predictor of ability to cope with living with HIV,

Elaine M. Hockman is affiliated with Wayne State University, Detroit, MI. Marcia Andersen and Geoffrey A. D. Smereck are affiliated with the Well-Being Institute, Detroit, MI.

Address correspondence to: Elaine M. Hockman, PhD, Coordinator, Research Support Laboratory, 10 Education Building, Wayne Sate University, Detroit, MI 48202 (E-mail: aa2073@wayne.edu).

This work was supported in part by the Health Resources and Services Administration (HRSA), HIV/AIDS Bureau (HAB), Special Projects of National Significance (SPNS) Grant No. BRU 900102-05. This publication's contents are solely the responsibility of the authors and do not necessarily represent the official view of the funding agency.

[Haworth co-indexing entry note]: "The Impact of an Intervention Program for HIV-Positive Women on Well-Being, Substance Use, Physical Symptoms, and Depression." Hockman, Elaine M., Marcia Andersen, and Geoffrey A. D. Smereck. Co-published simultaneously in *Drugs & Society* (The Haworth Press, Inc.) Vol. 16, No. 1/2, 2000, pp. 145-161; and: *Evaluating HIV/AIDS Treatment Programs: Innovative Methods and Findings* (ed: G. J. Huba et al.) The Haworth Press, Inc., 2000, pp. 145-161. Single or multiple copies of this article are available for a fee from The Haworth Document Delivery Service [1-800-342-9678, 9:00 a.m. - 5:00 p.m. (EST). E-mail address: getinfo@haworthpressinc.com].

and that depression was correlated with physical condition with respect to both status and change. *[Article copies available for a fee from The Haworth Document Delivery Service: 1-800-342-9678. E-mail address: <getinfo@haworthpressinc.com> Website: <http://www.HaworthPress.com>]*

KEYWORDS. HIV/AIDS, women, well-being, drug use, depression, nursing, evaluation

INTRODUCTION

HIV-positive women with a history of substance abuse are both a medically underserved population and an infrequent target of research. We know from the AIDS research literature, for example, that injection drug usage and unprotected sex put women at risk for contracting HIV and that risk is especially high among urban minorities. But little research has been reported on this population of women with respect to the course of the disease, treatment implications, psychosocial factors, and coping with the disease. From on-line searches of two databases, Current Contents Article Records and PsycINFO, using combinations of HIV, drugs, and well-being as search terms, we identified and retrieved 59 journal articles for thorough review after eliminating duplicate citations and multiple studies based upon the same samples. Of these 59 studies, only five, or 8%, dealt specifically with female HIV-positive populations; an additional 15% of these articles incorporated gender as a variable for analysis.

As part of an effort to reach underserved HIV-positive populations, the federal Health Resources and Services Administration (HRSA) has funded the Women's Intervention Program of the Well-Being Institute (WBI) to assist HIV-infected, substance-abusing women in accessing healthcare. WBI is a non-profit, community-based nursing organization in Detroit, Michigan.

The Personalized Nursing LIGHT Model

The WBI Women's Intervention Program stems from The Personalized Nursing LIGHT Model, an art of nursing model based on Martha Rogers' science of nursing (Rogers, 1986; Rogers, 1990). Dr. Rogers developed a science of nursing entitled the Science of Unitary Human Beings. The focus of any nursing intervention within this perspective is to assist the client to improve her sense of well-being toward a goal of reaching her maximum potential.

"Personalized Nursing" connotes the focus of care as being an individual's own identified *focal concerns*. Care is personalized to the person and the person's perception of what care is needed. Interventions are unique and creative to facilitate meeting the client's perceived needs. For example, nurses might make gravesite visits with grieving clients or provide dressings for wounds that need attention. Nurses do an individualized assessment and provide immediate care for the focal concerns of the moment that the client identifies. When clients are given attention and assistance with their focal concerns, they feel helped.

The Personalized Nursing model stresses that the path to optimal health and well-being lies within each person. Clients are given assistance and taught the LIGHT Model as a process to improve their sense of well-being, while remaining free of alcohol and drugs. An improved sense of well-being is associated with an ability to see more options and possibilities when confronted with life's problems and with a decrease in drug use and high risk sexual behaviors associated with AIDS acquisition and transmission (Andersen and Hockman, 1997).

The LIGHT Model, a symbol and acronym based on Florence Nightingale's lantern, gives direction to both the caregiver's role and the client's role in the healing process. The meanings of the acronym are outlined in Figure 1.

Bonding with Clients to Develop Trust

The first step of the intervention process is to bond with the client. The process of bonding or touching the client's soul requires the nurse to be alert

FIGURE 1. The LIGHT Model and Facets of the LIGHT Model Process

Nurses and Caregivers	Client
Love the client	Love yourself
Intend to help	Identify a concern
Give care gently	Give yourself a goal
Help client improve well-being	Have confidence and help yourself
Teach the process	Take positive action
• Bonding	Love the client
	Intend to be helpful
	Give your care gently
• Assess well-being and identity barriers	Help the client improve his/her well-being
• Teach the LIGHT Model	Teach a healing process and help clients plan the first step to deliberate pattern change

for clues in the client's words, mannerisms, dress, and environment. Nowhere is nursing more of an art than here.

Experience teaches several techniques that may be useful. Some clients, those who turn inward with their pain, grief, or low self-esteem, may be reached through the nurse's *sharing* of his/her own personal life experiences. Another medium, which seems to work, is the nurse's use of *metaphors* or the arts to establish commonalty and touch the soul of the client. *Intuition* is another medium that quickly and effectively provides clues on how to touch a patient. Nurses should go with their "intuition" when using this as a medium for bonding. Another bonding medium is *action caring*, an action in which the nurse takes pains to help the client. This is especially true when the action is inconvenient to the nurse because it demonstrates value and speaks louder than words. Action caring may touch the client's soul more than talking.

Assessing Well-Being and Identifying Barriers

After bonding with clients, an important aspect of the LIGHT Model is to assess the client's well-being and help the client improve it. To assess global well-being, the nurse asks each client how she feels about her life as a whole and to rate it on the delighted to terrible scale developed by Andrews and Withey (1978).

In cases where a client is less than delighted with her life, the nurse asks, "Why?" The client's answer helps identify barriers to maximum well-being. Clients are not always aware of their barriers to well-being–but these barriers to well-being are often also barriers to obtaining healthcare.

In addition to helping clients identify and address painful areas in their lives and/or focal concerns (concerns of the immediate moment), the staff assist clients to identify their special talents. Experience has shown each client has a talent or area of expertise or interest. When that area or talent is pursued, it is associated with a positive feeling of well-being. Nurses and other staff encourage clients to pursue their talents and provide tools for the client (paper, paints, etc.) when possible. As clients see themselves as talented people, valued by staff, they begin to see themselves as women worthy of healthcare.

Teaching a Healing Process and Planning the First Step
to Deliberate Change

Change happens. Directed change is the goal (Rogers, personal communication). Improvement of well-being is associated with more available energy. Once clients feel a little better, they have the energy to take action to improve their well-being and direct the changes occurring in their lives. They also have the energy to make and keep healthcare appointments.

Many artistic techniques can be used to encourage clients to take action to improve their sense of well-being. These include: facilitating experiential learning, role playing; giving a client new information; demonstrating, teaching specific tangible things clients need to know to make changes in their lives; giving support as clients attempt to interact and behave in new ways; and noticing and promoting talents within clients. The possibilities are endless.

The use of these creative interventions assists clients to take actions to help themselves. Clients have the answers inside themselves to overcome their barriers to well-being and their concerns. Nurses help clients plan their first steps to address their concerns. Once clients experience this process of helping themselves, they can repeat the process with future concerns.

A more thorough presentation of the philosophy, model, assumptions, and mode of operation of WBI can be found in Andersen et al. (1999).

Purpose

As its name implies, WBI aims to improve global well-being which is considered basic to confronting life's problems, especially those associated with substance abuse and chronic illness. The WBI program addresses the individual needs of HIV-positive women who are also substance abusers. As women enrolled in the program, it became evident that they also demonstrated mental illness, and, in many cases, the mental illness was severe. Our participants are thus considered to be "multiply diagnosed." Needs ranged from obtaining medical care for physical health problems, to addressing substance abuse issues, to dealing with mental health problems. In addition to these major concerns, the basics of life–need for food, shelter, and clothing–further compounded participants' conditions.

The literature stresses the importance of the mental health of HIV-infected persons with particular attention paid to depression and well-being. Depression had been identified as a serious, common, and treatable condition among HIV-infected persons (Bartlett, 1998; Katz et al., 1996). Up to 20% of patients suffer from major depression at the time of their initial presentation. Depression concurrent with symptomatic AIDS commonly presents tell-tale clinical symptoms (Bartlett, 1998): depressed mood, decreased interest in activities and anhedonia (loss of pleasure in activities), significant weight loss or weight gain, insomnia or hypersomnia (particularly early morning insomnia), motor agitation or retardation, fatigue or loss of energy, generalized feelings of worthlessness or excess or inappropriate guilt, difficulty with concentration, recurrent thoughts of death, and a profound sense of not-well-being, disproportionate to the severity of current medical problems.

The literature, however, presents conflicting evidence with respect to the relationship between depression and physical symptoms. Some report no correlation between depression and disease progression (Lyketsos et al., 1996b; Davis et al., 1995; Rabkin et al., 1997; Krikorian et al., 1995; Goggin et al., 1997; Cohen and Herbert, 1996). Other studies have found depression to increase with disease progression (Satz et al., 1997; Brauchli et al., 1997; Rabkin et al., 1997; Lyketsos et al., 1996a; Singh et al., 1997). While, further, some studies conclude that there are discontinuous or complexly-linked associations between depressive symptoms and disease progression (O'Dell et al., 1996; Zorilla et al., 1996; Mayne et al.,1996). Yet another interpretation is that depression is an intervening factor in disease progression (Johnson et al., 1995; Linn et al., 1996).

In this paper we address a series of questions to evaluate the WBI program with respect to its short-term effects in the areas of well-being, physical symptoms, depression, substance use, and ability to cope. Based upon WBI goals as well as the literature on depression among HIV-infected persons, our questions for evaluation are:

1. Does well-being improve among program clients over the course of their participation in the WBI Women's Intervention Program?
2. Is depression related to the extent to which physical symptoms interfere with normal activity? Do depression and physical symptoms improve over the course of participation in the WBI Women's Intervention Program?
3. Does substance abuse status improve among program clients over the course of their participation in the WBI Women's Intervention Program? Does substance usage decrease as well-being increases?
4. Do well-being, substance use, depression, and physical symptoms predict capacity to cope with living with HIV?

METHODS

Participants

Fifty-five HIV-positive women with a history of crack and/or alcohol abuse were recruited into the program and actively participated for a minimum of six months. Their ages at intake ranged from 25 to 50, with an average age of 37.7 years and standard deviation of 5.9. All participants were minorities, with 98% African American and 2% Native American. Only 40% were at least a high school graduate. The majority, 56%, was single, 36% were previously partnered such as divorced or widowed, and the remaining 8% currently had a domestic partner. All were unemployed.

Program

Needs Assessment

After recruitment into the program, the woman's needs with respect to medical care access, basic needs of living, substance abuse, mental health and coping skills were assessed. Simultaneous to enrolling clients in primary care, the nurses addressed the women's substance abuse and mental health problems. The model posits that once clients feel they are *worthy* of medical care and *have the time and energy* to participate in healthcare, appointments for primary medical and mental healthcare can be made and will likely be kept. Earlier projects have demonstrated that bonding with project staff and attention to improvement of well-being and mental health must occur prior to or simultaneous with attempts at linking HIV-positive substance abusers to primary healthcare (Andersen, Hockman, and Smereck, 1996).

Services

After a woman's needs were assessed, ways of overcoming barriers to her care were identified. Then the woman was linked to her necessary services. Briefly, the strategies used by WBI nurses to enroll women in primary care include (a) counseling using the LIGHT Model to prepare clients to access care, (b) activities, such as phone calls, to connect women to care, (c) accompaniment services, (d) provision of transportation, and (e) provision of child care. Counseling sessions may be individual- or group-based. Sessions focused on relevant study issues including physical health, substance dependency, mental health, living with HIV/AIDS, and on personally relevant issues including housing, food, shelter, and legal problems. Special attention was given to follow-up with respect to health-related referrals.

Evaluation Design

The evaluation plan for the WBI program was designed to address two major requirements. The first requirement was for an evaluation that reflected the philosophy, aims and methodology of WBI's Personalized Nursing LIGHT Model. This requirement led to procedures that are commensurate with the individualized nature of the WBI program. These procedures employ an intra-individual approach to assess, woman by woman, the progress she will have made with respect to accessing primary care, improving her sense of well-being and decreasing her psychological distress, and dealing with her substance abuse issues. In this approach, each woman serves as her own control for assessing the significance of change in well-being, substance usage, psychological distress, and coping capacity.

The second requirement was for an evaluation that would follow more traditional lines of investigation to assess the overall impact of the WBI program. The four study questions presented in the introduction to this paper served as the guide for the evaluation presented below. These questions are of global importance to HIV/AIDS care providers and the clients they serve. The basic evaluation procedure employed is essentially a pre-post analysis that assessed the sample's aggregate progress after a six-month program participation period. We looked at the sample's change in well-being, depression, physical symptoms, and substance use and at the relationship of these characteristics with coping capacity. If the application of the LIGHT model has been successful, a significant improvement in sense of well-being is expected. In addition, the evaluation tests the model's prediction that substance use will decline with well-being improvement. As for the relationships between depression and physical symptoms, we have seen conflicting results reported in the literature. We therefore have investigated that relationship in our sample of HIV-positive women. In addition to predicting that substance use will decline with well-being improvement, the underlying model of the program also predicts that improvement in sense of well-being will lead to more successful coping with life's problems. These are the questions that provide the focus for the evaluation that follows.

Study Measures

As the WBI program was part of a national cooperative agreement, we used a battery of assessment modules common across sites to track individual progress over a six-month participation interval after baseline assessment. All modules except the well-being scale were provided by The Measurement Group.

Well-Being

Andrews and Withey (1978) originally developed the measure of well-being used in this study. The instrument for the current evaluation consisted of 16 of the original 20 items about satisfaction with various aspects of life. The client rated each aspect on how she felt about this aspect of her life, taking into account what has happened in the past year and what she expects in the near future. A 7-point scale, from "terrible" to "delighted," was used. Four of the 20 items, although asked, were deleted from analysis for this study population because of inapplicability to many in the sample. Two of these items dealt with one's employment; one, with one's children; and one, with satisfaction with one's sex life. Women completed the well-being scale at intake and at follow-up.

Depression

The measure of depression used in this program was an 8-item version of the CES-D (Melchior et al., 1993). The client rated each depressive symptom on a 4-point scale ranging from "rarely or none of the time" to "most of the time." The time frame for experiencing each symptom was the past week. Women completed the depression scale at intake and at follow-up.

Physical Symptoms

The measure of health status dealt with the extent each of ten physical symptoms interfered with normal activity during the past four weeks. It consisted of 10 items from the Medical Outcomes Study Short Form Health Survey (Bozzette et al., 1995). Each symptom was rated on a 6-point scale ranging from "did not have it at all" to interferes "extremely" with normal activity. The time frame was the past four weeks. Women completed the physical symptoms scale at intake and at follow-up. The symptom areas included: aches/fatigue/lightheadedness; fevers/chills/sweats; poor appetite/ weight loss; trouble with eyes or ears; nose/sinuses/headache; mouth/swallowing; nausea/vomiting/diarrhea; coughing/wheezing/chest pain; rash/itch/ herpes/skin trouble; and numbness/tingling/arm, leg pain. Two symptoms that deal with psychological distress (trouble concentrating and depression) were excluded from this index to avoid the potential for a spurious relationship between physical symptoms and the measure of depression.

Coping Capacity

At time of follow-up, staff rated each woman on five target behaviors necessary for dealing with her disease (Huba et al., 1996). The behaviors were rated on 5-point scales ranging from "poor" to "excellent." These behaviors were: activities of daily living; follow-through with referrals; ability to obtain transportation; ability to deal with barriers; and compliance with medical advice.

Drug Behaviors

At intake, the women indicated their areas of substance use (Huba et al., 1997). For alcohol, the response categories were "today" if she had used it today or someone close to her thinks she has a problem with alcohol today; "current" if she or someone close to her thinks she has had a problem with alcohol in the last 30 days; "ever" if she or someone close to her thinks she has had a problem with alcohol in the past; and "never" if she or someone close to her thinks she has never had a problem with alcohol. For crack and heroin, the responses reflect her current usage: today, in the past 30 days, ever, and never. Indices of substance use were constructed from these responses to indicate whether the woman had used these substances within the past 30 days of intake and again within the past 30 days of follow-up.

Analysis Procedures

Scoring the Tests–Status at Intake and Follow-Up

The mean item response for the indices of Well-Being, Depression, and Coping Capacity were used instead of the simple sums of responses. This procedure has several useful properties. First, it handled the problem of occasional missing data. Less than 2% of scored items, however, were omitted in our sample. Simple sums underestimate a score in the case of missing data. Substitution of the sample's mean for a missing item response would introduce a bias in that the sample item variance would be reduced by a factor of $(n1 - 1)/(n - 1)$, where $n1$ is the number of cases answering the item and n is the total number of cases (Rubin, 1987). The second useful property in using the mean item response is that it gives an anchor for interpreting the means on the basis of the original item scale definitions, a characteristic especially useful in the absence of standard scores and norms. For example, a mean of "2" on Coping Capacity corresponds to a rating of "fair" in terms of the original item responses. When no items are missing, scores based on the average item response give identical statistical results as scores based on the sum of the ratings. By taking the average item response, we maximized the number of cases for analysis without imputing values for missing data. For Physical Symptoms we used the sum of the item responses, as these items are reflective of frequency.

Statistical Analyses

Reliabilities at intake and follow-up (Cronbach's coefficient alpha) as well as test-retest correlations and reliabilities of difference (change) scores were computed for Well-Being, Depression, and Physical Symptoms. Only cases with complete item responses were used in the calculations of the reliabilities. Intercorrelations among intake measures, follow-up measures, and change scores were computed. Paired t-tests (t-tests for correlated samples) were computed between intake and follow-up measures to assess significance of change to answer the questions of whether Well-Being improved and Depression and Physical Symptoms decreased from intake to follow-up. Because we wanted to evaluate change and how change related to outcome status, we computed the reliabilities of the difference scores. The McNemar chi-squared for correlated proportion (McNemar, 1962) was used to assess change in substance use status from intake to follow-up. Multiple regression analysis was used to predict Coping Capacity from Well-Being, Depression, Physical Symptoms, and change in substance use.

RESULTS

Psychometric Properties of the Study Measures

Internal consistency reliabilites (coefficient alpha) were computed for intake and follow-up measures of Well-Being, Depression, and Physical Symptoms. Test-retest reliabilities and reliabilities of the difference scores were also computed. These latter reliabilities are crucial for assessing and understanding change. Strong reliability of difference scores, a fundamental measure of change, is obtained when both initial and final reliabilities are high and test-retest correlation is low. For Well-Being, the intake reliability was

.87; follow-up, .88; test-retest, .42; and difference scores, .78. For Depression, the intake reliability was .83; follow-up, .92; test-retest, .34; and difference scores, .82. For Physical Symptoms, the intake reliability was .83; follow-up, .83; test-retest, .56; and difference scores, .62. The internal consistency reliability for Coping Capacity was .74.

For each of the three major study measures, the reliability of the difference scores was greater than the stability coefficient (test-retest reliability). Reliable difference scores are obtained when the reliabilities for the test and the retest are strong and the test-retest correlation is low (Lord, 1963; Hockman, 1971). That change from intake to follow-up had indeed occurred in our sample is evidenced by the strong reliabilities of the difference scores.

Changes in Sample Means from Intake to Follow-Up

The mean intake Well-Being item-response, 4.10, is at the mid-point of the Well-Being scale, defined as "mixed." For Depression, the mean intake item-response, 2.46, falls half-way between "some or a little of the time" and "occasionally." Using t-tests for correlated samples to assess total sample changes in Well-Being, Depression, and Physical Symptoms from intake to follow-up, we found that only Well-Being showed significant mean change from intake to follow-up. The change represented a significant improvement in sense of well-being. Although not significant, the changes in Depression and Physical Symptoms were in the hypothesized direction, a lessening of depression and physical symptoms. These findings are presented in Table 1.

Relationship Between Depression Change and Symptoms Change

Depression and Physical Symptoms measures were significantly correlated both at intake ($r = .50, p < .001$) and at follow-up ($r = .41, p = .005$). In addition, change in Depression was significantly correlated with change in Physical Symptoms ($r = .49, p = .004$). In contrast, Well-Being change was not significantly correlated with Depression change ($r = -.28, p = .081$) nor with Physical Symptoms ($r = -.009, p = .962$).

Substance Usage

Intake Assessment of Substance Problems

Although nearly every one had used alcohol at some time in the past, 32% considered alcohol a current problem at intake; 36% considered it a past problem; and 32% considered alcohol never a problem. As was found for alcohol, nearly everyone had used crack at some time in the past. However, in contrast to alcohol, crack usage was more frequently considered a problem: 46%, a problem in the past; 48%, a current problem; and 6%, never a prob-

TABLE 1. Mean Change in Well-Being, Depression, and Symptoms from Intake to Follow-Up

Measure	Well-Being	Depression	Symptoms
Intake			
Mean	4.10	2.46	18.1
SD	.986	.827	11.07
1st Follow-Up			
Mean	4.42	2.29	17.8
SD	.963	.915	10.24
Mean Change	.322	−.170	−.282
N	50	44	39
Paired *t*	2.416	1.121	167
p	.019	.268	868

lem. More than half the sample had used heroin at some time (59%). At intake, 10% considered heroin to be a current problem; 49% considered it a past problem; and 41% reported that they had never used it.

Change in Substance Usage

The percentages of women using alcohol and crack decreased from intake to follow-up. The decline in alcohol usage was significant (McNemar chi-squared for correlated proportions = 7.12, $p < .05$). The decline in crack usage was not significant. The current (past 30 days) usage percentages for alcohol, crack, and heroin are presented in Table 2.

Predicting Change in Substance Usage

Women were classified according to change in substance usage as either (a) "improving," i.e., using alcohol, crack, and/or heroin less at follow-up than at intake or (b) "not improving," i.e., showing no change or an increase in substance use from intake to follow-up. The WBI model predicts that substance usage decline will be associated with an improved sense of well-being. To test this association, repeated measures analyses of variance were computed with Well-Being, Depression, and Physical Symptoms as the repeated measures and substance usage status as the between-subjects factor.

TABLE 2. Change in Substance Usage from Intake to Follow-Up

Substance	% Using at Intake	% Using at Follow-Up	% Change
Alcohol	54.3%	30.4%	− 23.9%*
Crack	42.2%	26.7%	− 15.6%
Heroin	8.9%	11.1%	2.2%

Note. *Chi-square for correlated proportions = 7.12, p < .05

Results were as predicted for Well-Being. There was significant change from intake to follow-up ($F(1,40) = 5.68$, $p = .022$) and a significant interaction between the "time" (within-subjects) factor and substance usage status ($F(1,40) = 4.12$, $p = .049$). Improvement in well-being was significantly greater for those whose substance usage improved. There were no significant results for Depression or Physical Symptoms. Intake and follow-up means by substance use change category are presented in Table 3 for Well-Being, Depression, and Physical Symptoms.

Capacity to Cope as a Function of Well-Being, Physical Symptoms, and Change in Depression

A long-term goal of the WBI project is to enable clients to cope with life's problems. To assess initial progress toward this goal after approximately six months in the program, a multiple regression was computed to predict Coping Capacity from concurrent Well-Being, Physical Symptoms, Depression, and change in substance use. Individually, each of the measures was significantly associated with Coping Capacity: Well-Being, $r = .48$; Substance Use, $r = −.32$; Physical Symptoms, $r = −.28$; Depression, $r = −.27$. Looking at all measures simultaneously in a multiple regression, a significant prediction equation was found ($R = .55$, $p = .020$). However, Well-Being was the only measure that contributed significantly to the equation. The standardized regression coefficients are presented in Table 4.

DISCUSSION AND CONCLUSIONS

Individualized intervention for clients drawn from a population of HIV-positive women who have a history of substance abuse and mental health problems can effect positive, important changes to assist these women in

TABLE 3. Relationship Between Change in Substance Use and Change in Well-Being, Depression, and Physical Symptoms

Substance Usage Status at Follow-Up	Measure	Measure Means		
		Intake	Follow-Up	Change
Improved	Well-Being	4.13	4.75	.62*
Did Not Improve		4.11	4.17	.06
Improved	Depression	2.38	2.11	−.27
Did Not Improve		2.65	2.34	−.31
Improved	Physical Symptom	17.05	15.30	−1.75
Did Not Improve		20.50	18.86	−1.64

Note. *Within Subjects $F(1,40) = 5.68$, $p = .022$;
Interaction $F(1,40) = 4.12$, $p = .049$

TABLE 4. Summary of Regression Analysis Predicting Coping Capacity from Well-Being, Physical Symptoms, Depression, and Substance Use Change ($N = 37$)

Measure	β	t	p
Well-Being	.393	2.152	.039
Change in Substance Use	−.222	1.454	.156
Physical Symptoms	−.154	.954	.347
Depression	.027	.148	.883

Note. $R^2 = .30$, $F(4,32) = 3.390$, $p = .020$

coping with their life situation. The interventions provided by the WBI nurses and other staff are tailored to improve client well-being. Our data from intake and follow-up after six months in the program have shown that the program is working.

The treatment model employed by WBI, the Personalized Nursing LIGHT Model, postulates that improved well-being precedes positive change in important areas such as substance use and coping with chronic disease. The results of this evaluation after six months in the program demonstrate that (1) well-being has been positively impacted by the WBI intervention, (2) improvement in substance use is positively related to improvement in well-being, and (3) capacity to cope–with respect to every day activities, follow-through on referrals, obtaining transportation, dealing with barriers, and complying with medical advice–is positively related to well-being.

WBI staff work within the LIGHT model with each and every client to improve her sense of well-being. As a good model should, it provides a framework within which to work, but the methods and details of dealing with individual personalities, problems, and situations vary from client to client. The unique circumstances and characteristics of each client influence the direction her treatment will take. The staff need good judgment, flexibility, and a myriad of strategies to draw upon. Whatever the specific tact used with a client, the goal of improving the client's well-being remains constant. The theory behind the model states that an improved sense of well-being is associated with ability to see more options and possibilities when confronted with life's problems. These options include dealing with life without a dependency upon drugs. Our evaluation has shown that decrease in drug use was indeed associated with improvement in well-being.

As in the literature we reviewed, our data also show that the relationship between depression and physical symptoms is complex. We found that depression decreased as problems from physical symptoms decreased and depression increased as interference from physical symptoms increased. However, when problems from physical symptoms remain infrequent, depression also tends to remain constant at a low level. When problems from physical symptoms remained frequent, depression also tended to remain constant at a high level. Given that some participants increased on these measures, some decreased, and some remained constant, a lack of statistically significant change from intake to follow-up would be expected. This situation, of reliable but differential change, represents a major reason why we plan to extend our evaluation of the WBI program into the realm of intra-individual change measures. An intra-individual strategy will allow us to study the vicissitudes of change from individuals' points of view, which will reflect the "personalized" aspects of the WBI intervention and its impacts.

REFERENCES

Andersen, M. D. & Hockman, E. M. (1997). Well-being and high-risk drug use among active drug users. *Patterns of Rogerian Knowing* (chap. 13). New York: NLN Press.

Andersen, M. D., Hockman, E. M., & Smereck, G. A. D. (1996). Effect of a nursing outreach intervention to drug users in Detroit, Michigan. *Journal of Drug Issues*, *26*, 619-634.

Andersen, M. D., Smereck, G. A. D., Hockman, E. M., Ross, D. J., & Ground, K. J. (1999). Nurses decrease barriers to healthcare by "hyperlinking" multiple-diagnosed women living with HIV/AIDS into care. *Journal of the Association of Nurses in AIDS Care, 10*, 55-65.

Andrews, F. M. & Withey, S. B. (1978). *Social indicators of well-being.* New York: Plenum.

Bartlett, J. G. (1998). *Medical management of HIV infection.* Baltimore, MD: Johns Hopkins University Division of Infectious Diseases.

Bozzette, S. A., Hays, R. D., Wu, A. W., Berry, S. H., & Kanouse, D. (1995). Derivation and psychometric properties of a brief health-related quality of life instrument for HIV disease. *Journal of Acquired Immunodeficiency Syndromes and Retrovirology, 8,* 253-265.

Brauchli, P. & Zeier, H. (1997). Depression and immune status in HIV-infected persons. *Psychotherapie Psychosomatik Medizinische Psychology, 47,* 34-40.

Cohen, S. & Herbert, T. B. (1996). Health psychology: Psychological factors and physical disease from the perspective of human psychoneuroimmunology. *Annual Review of Psychology, 47,* 113-142.

Davis, K. J., Metzger, D. S., Meyers, K., McLellan, R. T., Mulvaney, F. D., Navaline, H. A., & Woody, G. E. (1995). Long-term changes in psychological symptomatology associated with HIV serostatus among male injecting drug users. *AIDS, 9,* 73-79.

Goggin, K. J., Zisook, S., Heaton, R. K., Atkinson, J. H., Marshall, S., McCutchan, J. A., Chandler, J. L., & Grant, I. (1997). Neuropsychological performance of HIV-1 infected men with major depression. *Journal of International Neuropsychology & Sociology, 3,* 457-464.

Hockman, E. M. (1971). *The validation of interindividual and intra-individual change measures.* Unpublished doctoral dissertation, University of Michigan, Ann Arbor.

Huba, G. J., Melchior, L. A., Staff of The Measurement Group, and the HRSA SPNS Program Cooperative Agreement Projects (1997). *Module 1: Demographic Contact Form.* Available: www.TheMeasurementGroup.com. Culver City, California: The Measurement Group.

Huba, G. J., Melchior, L. A., Staff of The Measurement Group, and the HRSA SPNS Program Cooperative Agreement Projects (1996). *Module 42: Psychosocial Observations Form.* Available: www.TheMeasurementGroup.com. Culver City, California: The Measurement Group.

Johnson, J. G., Williams, J. B., Rabkin, J. G., Goetz, R. R., & Remien, R. H. (1995). Axis I psychiatric symptoms associated with HIV infection and personality disorder. *American Journal of Psychiatry, 152,* 551-554.

Katz, M. H., Douglas, J. M., Bolan, G. A., Marx, R., Sweat, M., Park, M. S., & Buchbinder, S. P. (1996). Depression and use of mental health services among HIV-infected men. *AIDS Care, 8,* 433-442.

Krikorian, R., Kay, J., & Lian, W. M. (1995). Emotional distress, coping, and adjustment in human immunodeficiency virus infection and acquired immune deficiency syndrome. *Journal of Nervous & Mental Disease, 183,* 293-298.

Linn, J. G., Anema, M. G., Hodess, S., Sharpe, C., & Cain, V. A. (1996). Perceived health, HIV illness, and mental distress in African-American clients of AIDS counseling centers. *Journal of the Association of Nurses in AIDS Care, 7,* 43-51.

Lord, F. M. (1963). Elementary models for measuring change. In Harris, C. W. (Ed.),

Problems in measuring change (pp. 21-38). Madison: The University of Wisconsin Press.

Lyketsos C. G., Hoover, D. A., Guccione, M., Dew, M. A., Wesch, J. E., Bing, E. G., & Treisman, G. J. Changes in depressive symptoms as AIDS develops. (1996a). *American Journal of Psychiatry, 153*, 1430-1437.

Lyketsos, C. G., Hoover, D. A., Guccione, M., Dew, M. A., Wesch, J. E., Bing, E. G., & Treisman, G. J. (1996b). Depressive symptoms over the course of HIV infection before AIDS. *Social Psychiatry and Psychiatric Epidemiology, 31*, 212-219.

Mayne, T. J., Vittinghoff, E., Chesney, M. A., Barrett, D. C., & Coates, T. J. (1996). Depressive affect and survival among gay and bisexual men infected with HIV. *Archives of Internal Medicine, 156*, 2233-2238.

McNemar, Q. (1962). *Psychological statistics (3rd Ed)*. New York: Wiley.

Melchior, L. A., Huba, G. J., Brown, V. B., & Reback, C. J. (1993). A short depression index for women. *Educational and Psychological Measurement, 53*, 1117-1125.

O'Dell, M. W., Meighen, M., & Riggs, R. V. (1996). Correlates of fatigue in HIV infection prior to AIDS: A pilot study. *Disability Rehabilitation, 18*, 249-254.

Rabkin, J. G., Goetz, R. R., Remien, R. H., Williams, J. B., Todak, G., & Gorman, J. M. (1997). Stability of mood despite HIV illness progression in a group of homosexual men. *American Journal of Psychiatry, 154*, 231-238.

Rogers, M. E. (1986). Science of unitary human beings. In V. Malinski (Ed.), *Explorations on Martha Rogers' science of unitary human beings*. Norwalk, CT: Appleton-Century-Crofts.

Rogers, M. E. (1990). Nursing: Science of unitary irreducible, human beings: Update 1990. In E. A. M. Barrett (Ed.), *Visions of Rogers' science-based nursing* (pp. 5-11). New York: NLN Press.

Rubin, D. B. (1987) *Multiple Imputation for Nonresponse in Surveys*. New York: Wiley.

Satz, P., Myers, H. F., Maj, M., Fawzy, F., Forney, D. L., Bing, E. G., Richardson, M. A., & Janssen, R. (1997). Depression, substance use, and sexual orientation as cofactors in HIV-1 infected men: Cross-cultural comparisons. *NIDA Research Monograph, 172*, 130-155.

Singh, N., Squier, C., Sivek, C., Wagener, M. M., & Yu, V. L. (1997). Psychological stress and depression in older patients with intravenous drug use and human immunodeficiency virus infection: implications for intervention. *International Journal of STD & AIDS, 8*, 251-255.

Zorilla E. P., McKay, J. R., Luborsky, L., & Schmidt, K. (1996). Relation of stressors and depressive symptoms to clinical progression of viral illness. *American Journal of Psychiatry, 153*, 626-635.

Practical Issues
in Evaluating a Self-Structured
Psychosocial and Medical Support Program
for Women with HIV/AIDS:
PROTOTYPES WomensLink,
a Community-Based Organization

Lisa A. Melchior, PhD
Chi Hughes, MSW
Vivian B. Brown, PhD
G. J. Huba, PhD

SUMMARY. PROTOTYPES WomensLink was developed to meet the needs of women living with HIV in greater Los Angeles, California. At the WomensLink drop-in center, women select the program components in which to participate, reflecting their unique medical and psy-

Lisa A. Melchior and G. J. Huba are affiliated with The Measurement Group, Culver City, CA. Chi Hughes and Vivian B. Brown are affiliated with PROTO-TYPES, Culver City, CA.

Address correspondence to: Lisa A. Melchior, PhD, Vice President, The Measurement Group, 5811A Uplander Way, Culver City, CA 90230 (E-mail: lmelchior@ TheMeasurementGroup.com).

This work was supported in part by the Health Resources and Services Administration (HRSA), HIV/AIDS Bureau (HAB), Special Projects of National Significance (SPNS) Grant No. 5 U90 HA 00030-05. The contents of this publication are solely the responsibility of the authors and do not necessarily represent the official view of the funding agency.

[Haworth co-indexing entry note]: "Practical Issues in Evaluating a Self-Structured Psychosocial and Medical Support Program for Women with HIV/AIDS: PROTOTYPES WomensLink, a Community-Based Organization." Melchior, Lisa A. et al. Co-published simultaneously in *Drugs & Society* (The Haworth Press, Inc.) Vol. 16, No. 1/2, 2000, pp. 163-184; and: *Evaluating HIV/AIDS Treatment Programs: Innovative Methods and Findings* (ed: G. J. Huba et al.) The Haworth Press, Inc., 2000, pp. 163-184. Single or multiple copies of this article are available for a fee from The Haworth Document Delivery Service [1-800-342-9678, 9:00 a.m. - 5:00 p.m. (EST). E-mail address: getinfo@haworthpressinc.com].

chosocial needs. Although this service model poses a number of challenges to program evaluation, including those related to evaluation design and implementation, it presents new opportunities for successful collaborations between community-based programs and applied researchers. This paper discusses a number of such issues and provides selected evaluation results that demonstrate the success of the Womens-Link model in meeting its goals of caring for women living with HIV and their families. *[Article copies available for a fee from The Haworth Document Delivery Service: 1-800-342-9678. E-mail address: <getinfo@haworthpress inc.com> Website: <http://www.HaworthPress.com>]*

KEYWORDS. Women, HIV/AIDS, community-based organization, program evaluation, substance abuse

INTRODUCTION

Across the nation, women are the fastest growing group of persons with HIV (CDC, 1999). As the number of women living with HIV/AIDS has grown over the course of the epidemic and continues to escalate (Campbell, 1999), innovative service delivery models have been developed to meet the needs of the women and their families. The most promising of these models provide integrated services that are individualized, using a client-centered approach (e.g., Brown, Hughes, Melchior, & Huba, 1998; Stober, Schwartz, McDaniel, & Abrams, 1997) that emphasize methods that will help the woman obtain timely care for her medical and psychosocial needs (e.g., Siegel, Karus, & Raveis, 1997) while reducing barriers to accessing such care (e.g., Raveis, Siegel, & Gorey, 1998; Russell & Smith, 1998). PROTO-TYPES developed its WomensLink program for women with HIV/AIDS and their families to provide a drop-in, client-driven service model in which the women choose from a wide array of services to participate in those interventions that best meet their unique needs.

Evaluation of community-based service demonstration projects, such as the WomensLink program for women living with HIV/AIDS, is essential for documenting the achievements of these innovative service models, and to provide a model for replicating the program in other contexts (Huba, Brown, Melchior, Hughes, & Panter, this volume). However, the evaluation of such programs involves a number of practical issues that can affect the design, implementation, and ultimately, outcomes of applied evaluation research in this setting. In community-based programs such as this one, traditional "textbook" evaluation methods may not be appropriate or otherwise fall short of producing an evaluation that adequately demonstrates the outcomes achieved by the program (Huba & Melchior, 1996). This paper describes several such practical issues encountered in designing and implementing the evaluation of the PROTOTYPES WomensLink program. We also present a number of strategies we have found to be helpful in measuring the progress of the program in achieving its goals, objectives, and desired outcomes.

The Need for Woman-Sensitive HIV Services in Los Angeles, California

HIV/AIDS continues to disproportionately affect women, especially women of color (CDC, 1999; Los Angeles County Department of Health Services, 1999). Although many treatment advances have created tremendous promise for people living with HIV/AIDS in recent years, those groups traditionally underserved by the healthcare system and who have had limited access to quality healthcare have not fully benefited from these advances. In addition, these groups have encountered a number of barriers to maximizing their use of healthcare resources in the community. In response to the growing need for psychosocial and medical support services for women living with HIV/AIDS, PROTOTYPES WomensLink was developed in 1994.

The need for woman-sensitive HIV services in the greater Los Angeles area is immense. As of June 1999, Los Angeles County had more than 39,000 cumulative AIDS cases, second in the US only to New York City (Los Angeles County Department of Health Services, 1999). In the last five years, *women have become the fastest growing population at-risk for HIV/AIDS*, with alarming increases occurring among African American women and Latinas. The epidemiology of HIV/AIDS among women in Los Angeles is similar to that found nationally. As of June 30, 1999, there were more than 2,600 women in Los Angeles County documented to have AIDS, with the majority (75 percent) being women of color (Los Angeles County Department of Health Services, 1999). To meet the needs of this population, PROTOTYPES conducts intensive outreach to women of color in minority neighborhoods in the hopes of bringing them into a service system specifically designed for their unique needs.

PROTOTYPES WomensLink was created to help address the insensitivity frequently found in traditional systems of disease prevention, healthcare, and treatment with respect to women, particularly substance abusers. Clients in this setting are often labeled as "non-compliant," difficult, too much trouble, disruptive, mistrustful, and manipulative. WomensLink was developed to help empower women living with HIV/AIDS to navigate through these potentially difficult healthcare systems and to advocate for the needs of themselves and their families. Women living with HIV confront a number of difficulties in accessing care, including being forced to "fit" into a system designed to serve gay and bisexual men (e.g., Rosen & Blank, 1992), facing difficulties obtaining public assistance benefits, lacking child care at HIV service agencies, finding day care and respite services, locating adoption services to help mothers near death make adoption arrangements for their children, lacking information about special "family" services, such as family menus at food bank services, insensitivity to substance abusers, and having long waits for services. For women living with HIV who are also substance abusers, the number of unmet service needs may be even greater and service access can be especially difficult (e.g., Weissman & Brown, 1996; Weissman, Melchior, Huba, Smereck, Needle, McCarthy, Jones, Genser, Cottler, Booth, & Altice, 1995). In light of findings that fewer women than men tend to receive assistance in linking to care upon first learning of a positive HIV test, especially with respect to medical services (Huba & Melchior, 1994; Weissman, Melchior, Huba, Altice, Booth, Cottler, Genser, Jones, McCarthy, Needle, & Smereck, 1995), the need for help in making such connections seems especially critical.

The PROTOTYPES WomensLink Model

PROTOTYPES WomensLink is a tightly linked, comprehensive, progressive continuum of medical, mental health and social services for women affected by and living with HIV/AIDS. Key to this concept is a storefront meeting place where women and their families can congregate to receive guidance and counseling, avail themselves of professional and peer supportive services, learn about and be linked to resources, and receive opportunities for socialization–all too often lacking due to isolation resulting from the stigma of AIDS. This approach thus involves a program focusing on the complex inter-related needs of women, their children and families; centralized outreach and intake services for substance abusing women, particularly active users; direct linkage of women via strong case management to a broad array of professional and peer-directed services; inclusion of persons with HIV/AIDS in planning for and provision of service delivery; culturally appropriate, culturally competent programs, staff and volunteers; development of a collaborative *settlement house* model of service provision; and training for primary care providers to increase knowledge, receptivity and skill in treating substance abusing women.

Based on these concepts, PROTOTYPES developed WomensLink, a multi-cultural and collaborative model of service delivery bringing together a broad array of resources for women. It is based upon the *settlement house* model of community-based services, in which underserved and disenfranchised individuals, families, and communities are afforded the opportunity to become empowered through a grass-roots approach involving *helpers* from the community in which they live. Elements of this model popularized by social reformer Jane Addams of Chicago's Hull House are used in the WomensLink program.

The WomensLink facility, a community-based resource, is designed around the woman: her specific medical and health needs, her barriers to accessing care, her family and her relationships. Any woman living with HIV/AIDS in Los Angeles County is eligible to benefit from the services provided by the culturally sensitive staff of PROTOTYPES and its cooperating agencies. Women living with HIV/AIDS are assisted in accessing services through interventions that reduce barriers such as providing transportation and childcare, while increasing the women's skills in interacting with service providers and the provider's skill in interacting with the women.

At WomensLink, clients are linked to a number of continuing care services through a collaboration of internal and external resources. Figure 1 shows the flow of women through the program. Women are recruited through a series of outreach activities conducted by PROTOTYPES staff under various local, state, and federal contracts and grants. Several thousand women a year are contacted and screened through these programs that operate in some of the poorest neighborhoods of Los Angeles County. All women linked to the outreach process receive a needs assessment for HIV services, and if they test positive and wish services are then moved into service options appropriate to their biopsychosocial needs. Women whose primary need is greater than what can be provided in community-based outpatient services for HIV may be moved into PROTOTYPES services offered for substance abuse and mental health problems, which are more intensive modalities of treatment for multiply diagnosed women. Clients are also referred to WomensLink by other HIV service providers, clinics, hospitals, the Department of Children and Family Services, the criminal justice system, and family members.

Evaluating the WomensLink Model

Recognizing that evaluability would be a key to the success of WomensLink as a national service demonstration model, program and evaluation elements were integrated from the project's inception. In general, the program evaluation addresses four broad questions: (1) Who is served by the program? (2) What services does the program provide? (3) How does the model work? and (4) What outcomes are associated with participating in the WomensLink program? However, there are a number of issues that arise in designing and implementing the evaluation of a community-based consumer-driven program such as this one. The following questions must be addressed in the evaluation of such programs.

Issues from the Program Perspective

Who collects evaluation data? The evaluation design (p. 172) specifies that program staff members collect much of the process and outcome data. Reasons for this include the fact that the clients are likely to build a rapport

FIGURE 1. Overview of Health Services Continuum in PROTOTYPES WomensLink

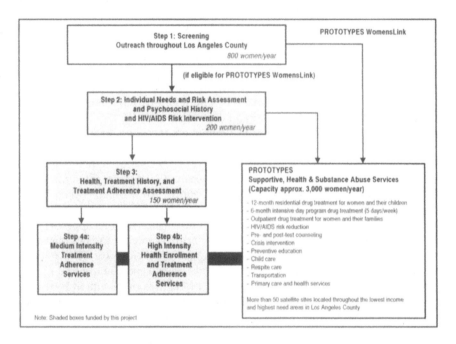

with staff over time, and consequently may provide more valid data. In addition, staff document services provided to the women as they provide them to the client (or shortly thereafter), again improving the reliability of the data. Much of the data collected for program evaluation are needed for other clinical or data reporting (e.g., to alternate funding sources) purposes and therefore reduces burden on the women. In a service demonstration project such as this one, it must also be recognized that funding levels for data collection are not the same as in a traditional research project; thus having staff serve multiple roles helps to provide the most efficient use of resources for evaluation data collection.

However, there are some tradeoffs in using program staff for this purpose (see also Huba, Brown, Melchior, Hughes, & Panter, this volume). The multidisciplinary, multicultural WomensLink staff members are primarily clinicians, not researchers. Because they are collecting evaluation data as part of their daily activities, they may be cast in dual roles: those of clinician and data collector. It may also be difficult at times for clients to make the distinction. One way we have attempted to distinguish evaluation from program activities is to provide incentives for participation in evaluation activities that exceed the level of data collection and documentation that are normally part of clinical record-keeping, client assessment, and tracking of individual client progress. As a team, program managers, staff, and evaluators have worked hard to maintain the boundaries and differentiate usual programmatic activities from those related to program evaluation and research.

Finally, certain outcome data collection activities, such as conducting follow-up interviews and chart reviews are conducted by professional evaluators rather than program staff. In such instances, the objectivity of an outside evaluator is highly desirable in reviewing archival documents (such as client charts) or in asking women to reflect back on their involvement with the program (such as in follow-up interviews).

How integrated should program and evaluation activities be? Despite concerns about blending program and evaluation activities, some program events may be used as incentives for clients to participate in both program and evaluation activities. For example, to increase response rates for a follow-up study of program participants, WomensLink held a number of special events to bring women who had not recently accessed services back to the program. The events provided additional opportunities for therapeutic and social contact with the women while also creating an opportunity to participate in outcome evaluation data collection. Despite these creative solutions, however, it can be a challenge to optimize the relative integration of program and evaluation issues.

How will clients react to evaluation procedures? The expectation of women who enroll in services at WomensLink is that they will receive supportive services related to HIV/AIDS. They are not necessarily seeking the experience of participating in a research study. One of the major challenges of designing and implementing a program evaluation in this setting is to make the data collection as unobtrusive as possible, maximize the clinical utility of the evaluation data, while at the same time ensuring that the client's needs are met as the first priority.

How will the program use the evaluation data? Program managers have found the availability of data reports on service utilization patterns, staff productivity, and other program trends to be useful. In the case of WomensLink, a monthly management information report is generated by the evaluation team and provided to program mangers to review service delivery patterns at the program level. We have found that the ability to produce such management information reports from evaluation data is useful for keeping program managers informed and providing a short-term use of the data. Although the primary purpose of the evaluation is to address "big picture" questions about process and outcomes of the service delivery model, the ability to address continuing quality assurance concerns is also an important function of program evaluation in this setting.

Issues from the Evaluation Perspective

What is the best way to evaluate a program in which each woman receives an individualized set of services? As a drop-in program, clients may attend services at WomensLink when they want; as a result, some may come in sporadically, while others may have relatively intensive involvement with the program. Because the program's services are highly individualized and self-selected by the client, a traditional "fixed" evaluation design is not practical. As a related point, it was recognized early in the design of the WomensLink program and its evaluation that examining service utilization patterns would be key to understanding the model, as well as predicting client outcomes. "Dosage" or intensity of program involvement was identified as a useful proxy measure of "engagement" in care that would likely be related to a number of intermediate and long-term outcomes for the clients and the program as a whole. Thus, the evaluation design adopted for WomensLink utilized measures of program involvement, as well as measures of health and psychosocial outcomes.

In addition to using indicators of program involvement to moderate the prediction of client outcomes, the actual measurement of such outcomes was addressed in a number of ways. First, because women do not visit the program at fixed intervals, a data collection "sweeps" strategy was used to collect certain outcome data. In the sweeps methodology, participants are sampled during a specified time period. In a given time period (in this case, a month), each client is administered a particular scale or procedure the first time she attends the program during the month. For instance, assume that we want to measure changes in psychological well-being over time. A pragmatic and practical way to do this is to administer a short measure of psychological functioning to each program participant the first time she is seen by the program in March, again in July, and again in November. If, in the same program, we wished to measure changes in perceived barriers to care, we could give a short assessment the first time the program sees the participants in February, June, and October. From the standpoint of staff, time-bound sampling is desirable because each month they do a special form, or forms, when they first see a client, thus minimizing data collection burden at any given time. Analytically, a "two-way" design is used to assess change in which one factor is "first administration, second administration, etc." (the repeated measure) and the other is the length of time the client was in the program when the outcome measure was administered. If analyzed in a traditional analysis of variance, the design is one in which the administration variable would be seen as a "random factor."

A second data collection methodology implemented in the WomensLink evaluation was that of a semi-structured follow-up interview. Collecting long-term outcome data in the sense of a "follow-up" was somewhat unusual in this setting, in that there was no set length of program involvement for clients, and that as a self-structured, drop-in program, clients do not necessarily "complete" or "drop out" of treatment. Yet it was very important from the evaluation perspective to collect long-term outcome data from the women so that the impact of the program could be demonstrated. To address these challenges, a follow-up methodology was implemented wherein women were eligible for follow-up six months after their initial program visit, whether or not they were still actively involved with the program at that time. In contrast to the data sweeps, which were integrated as part of the usual data collection activities of program staff, follow-up interviews were treated as a relatively independent data source. Evaluation staff conducted the follow-up interviews and small incentives were provided for the clients to participate in the follow-up "study."

Finally, utilization of chart review activities by the evaluation team allowed us to identify various issues in the client records that could not be collected through self-report or staff report and also permitted the collection of information from archival records that had not been originally anticipated. For example, when the program was originally designed, combination therapies using protease inhibitors had not yet come into use. Yet the availability of such treatments radically changed the face of HIV/AIDS treatment. To capture these important data, chart review procedures were developed to obtain relevant information from client records.

What domains should be measured to best evaluate client progress? Another challenge in evaluating the services demonstration program at WomensLink, as is true of evaluating many publicly funded community service programs, is that there are multiple issues to capture in terms of both process and outcome. Given that WomensLink is a multidisciplinary program addressing the various needs of its clients, the evaluation needed to be flexible enough to be able to capture a wide array of relevant issues, ranging from linking women with medical care and psychosocial supports including substance abuse treatment, to providing transportation and housing assistance. Yet at the same time, concerns about overburdening clients and staff limit the extent of data collection that is possible in this setting. As can be seen in the evaluation design for WomensLink, data concerning a wide array of health and psychosocial issues are collected in a relatively parsimonious way.

What is the ideal balance between local and cross-cutting evaluation concerns? Many federal health service initiatives are increasing their emphasis on multisite evaluation, given increased pressures from policy makers to be able to demonstrate effectiveness and cost-effectiveness of national service demonstration programs. In addition, those same initiatives require each service demonstration project to evaluate its own model ("local evaluation") to demonstrate the process and outcomes associated with a given service delivery model. Both program staff and evaluators were integrally involved in striking the balance and coordinating these two important concerns. While the program and evaluation were initially designed to maximize what could be demonstrated for WomensLink, the project was proposed knowing that there would be a cross-cutting evaluation, and that the local activities would need to mesh with the requirements of the multisite activities. However, the specific requirements of the cross-cutting evaluation were not known at the time the project was proposed and the local evaluation was designed. Thus it was necessary to anticipate a number of possible contingencies that the project and its evaluation would need to be able to accommodate once the cross-cutting evaluation elements were implemented. Even after beginning to develop the cross-cutting evaluation through a consensus-building process among 27 diverse grantees (see Huba, Melchior, Panter, Brown, & Larson, this volume), the parameters of the national evaluation could not be known until several months into the collective process.

Joining Program and Evaluation Perspectives

Although many of the questions raised above originate from programmatic or evaluation perspectives, the best solutions are likely to join the two points of view. In designing and implementing the evaluation of the Womens-Link model, program and evaluation issues have been linked at every step. Oversight for the evaluation is the responsibility of the evaluation team. While data entry and statistical analyses are conducted at the evaluator's offices, case managers and treatment staff collect evaluation data from clients as part of their responsibilities. The program staff/data collectors are also responsible for ensuring that information is regularly forwarded to the evaluators. All staff are trained in data collection on a regular basis by evaluation staff. The evaluation was designed so that information is collected that is also of vital importance to the program staff. Evaluation data are coded onto computer-usable forms not only for ongoing process evaluation, but also so that program managers can regularly receive management information reports to monitor program activities. The key to successful program-evaluation collaborations is to ensure that these activities occur on an ongoing basis.

Evaluation Design

To address the various concerns identified above, the following evaluation design was developed and implemented. As illustrated in Table 1, a variety of process and outcome issues are addressed in the various data elements collected throughout the clients' involvement in the program, using a blend of quantitative and qualitative methods.

TABLE 1. Ongoing Data Collection Forms in the WomensLink Program Evaluation

Form	Brief Description	Major Indicators	When Collected
Enrollment Form (Module 1)	Used to code major demographic characteristics of clients, risk-background factors, reason for completing the form, and referrals provided at contact.	Race/ethnicity, gender, sexual orientation, age, location, housing status, HIV infection-retransmission risk factors, and referral source.	• At intake • Updates as necessary
Daily Services Form (Module 2B)	Used to document psychosocial services provided to an individual on a particular day or during a specific contact episode.	Prevention/intervention services, mental health services, group counseling, substance abuse services, case management/advocacy services, topics discussed, and services provided by.	• Intake • Each visit
Barriers to Treatment (Module 4B)	Used to collect information on client perceptions of barriers and facilitators to services, and to identity perceived difficulty of clients obtaining services.	Barriers include: cost, accessibility, lack of transportation, lack of child care, perceived staff disdain, language, coercion, and disclosure concerns. Facilitators include: caring staff, child care, convenient location, and transportation.	• Intake • 3-month intervals
Client Satisfaction with Services (Module 11)	Used to code major aspects of satisfaction or dissatisfaction with services.	Overall ratings of satisfaction with services, perceptions of service providers, and recommendations regarding family/peer services.	• 3-month intervals
Health-Related Quality of Life (Module 17)	RAAD SF-21 (Bozzette, Hays, Wu, Berry, & Kanouse, 1995) includes eight functioning scales and a categorical health rating.	Client/patient functioning, utilization of healthcare services, financial resources and physical symptoms.	• Intake • 3-month intervals
Substance Abuse History (Module 24)	Collects information on alcohol and other drugs used during the person's lifetime, in the last six months, and in the last 30 days.	Age drugs were first used, whether drugs had ever been injected, age of first injection drug use.	• Intake • 3-month intervals
Center for Epidemiologic Studies Depression (CESD-8) (Module 26B)	Collects information about a client's level of psychological distress using an 8-item version of the CES-D (Melchior, Huba, Brown, & Reback, 1993).	Days in the last week that the client felt depressed, moody, lonely, fearful, and restless.	• Intake • 3-month intervals

TABLE 1 (continued)

Form	Brief Description	Major Indicators	When Collected
Referral Form (Module 51)	Used to track service referrals made to collateral and cooperating agencies.	Agencies include: HIV testing, STD clinics, medical emergencies, inpatient and outpatient medical/mental health services, social services, food/drop-in services, housing/shelters, educational/vocational training, self-help groups, case management, substance abuse treatment, family planning/support, legal services, child care, advocacy services, transportation, and alternative therapy.	• Each time a referral is made
Items Provided Form	Used to document items provided to the client during a service episode.	Membership packet, household/hygiene supplies, brochures, educational materials, referrals, wallet cards, immunizations, medications, condoms, dental dams, transportation, and food/vouchers.	• Each time an item is provided
Needs Form	Used to document services needed by women and to assist women with a variety of services and referrals.	Peer support, HIV 12-Step groups, counseling, family support, case management, advocacy/education, housing referrals, necessities canteen, food/vouchers, transportation, social activities, substance abuse treatment, and legal assistance.	• Intake • "Periodic" needs assessments
Hotline Form	Used to code client's calls to a hotline when such calls constitute a service. Also used to code referrals made to participating social service agencies.	Tracking of client characteristics and nature of call, referrals for social services, mental health, substance abuse treatment, and basic needs services.	• Each time call is logged
Discharge Form	Codes reasons for discharge.	Voluntary/involuntary withdrawal, referrals, moving away from service area, program completion, hospitalization, and death.	• When client is known to be "lost"
Follow-Up Interviews	To identify long-term medical and psychosocial outcomes of WomensLink clients	Linkages to medical services, linkages to social services, satisfaction with care compared to that obtained prior to program involvement, health status, service needs and how helpful the program was in addressing those needs, adherence and participation in HIV care, medication history and adherence issues, and linkages to services needed for children.	• Six months following enrollment, and at six month intervals thereafter
Chart reviews	To capture initial linkages to care upon entry to WomensLink, additional information regarding prescribed treatments, clinical issues, and related information	Additional information about intake (e.g., referral source, previous sources of HIV care), health indicators (e.g., CD4 count, viral load when available, history of opportunistic infections), medication history, psychiatric history, information about client's child(ren).	• Updated by evaluation staff periodically

Later in this paper we report selected outcomes from the PROTOTYPES WomensLink program as an example of the data "sweeps" methodology. The three measures used in these examples are described below.

Barriers to care. The Service Barriers and Facilitators Questionnaire (SBFQ) is a 28-item instrument used to measure perceived barriers to obtaining services and facilitators for receiving services. The SBFQ includes 17 items about service barriers and 11 for service facilitators. Each of the items is scored on a scale of 0 (the item was not a barrier/facilitator) to 1 (the item was a barrier/facilitator); a score of ".5" means that the woman did not know if the item was a barrier/facilitator. Total scores for (a) barriers and (b) facilitators are computed by summing the barrier item scores and by summing the facilitator item scores, respectively. The form is available on the Internet at www.TheMeasurementGroup.com/modules.htm. In the present context, the SBFQ was administered as a structured interview by program staff. Only the "barriers" data are reported here.

Psychological distress. The Center for Epidemiological Studies Depression Scale (CES-D) is a 20-item scale used to measure current psychological distress (Radloff, 1977). For this evaluation, a psychometrically sound, 8-item short version (Melchior et al., 1993; Huba et al., 1995) was used. The short form employed here is correlated .93 with the full instrument in a community sample of high-need women.

Service intensity. Services were coded using a standard instrument, the Psychosocial Services Module 2B (Huba et al., 1997b) which was implemented as part of the cross-cutting evaluation for the HRSA SPNS Cooperative Agreement Projects. This form is available on the Internet at www.TheMea surementGroup.com/modules.htm. The form captures the dates of services and the time expended in them in the categories of HIV Intervention Service Days, Mental Health Service Days, Group Counseling Service Days, Substance Abuse Service Days, and Case Management/Advocacy Service Days.

RESULTS

Evaluating the implementation of the model. By turning the conceptual flow chart shown in Figure 1 into measurable goals and objectives, it is possible to operationalize the steps in Figure 1 and evaluate the success of the program at achieving the desired flow of women through services. Table 2 shows the WomensLink program's goals, activities, and relevant evaluation issues and data.

Between 1994 and 1999, 404 women living with HIV/AIDS participated in services at PROTOTYPES WomensLink. The program reaches a diverse group of women, with 51.5 percent African American, 24.8 percent Latina, 17.6 percent Caucasian, 1.2 percent Asian American, 0.7 Native American,

TABLE 2. Selected Project Goals and Issues in Their Evaluation upon WomensLink Program Implementation

Original Goal	Operationalization	Relevant Evaluation Issues	Relevant Evaluation Data 1994-1999
Goal 1: To provide a range of quality services to targeted HIV-infected, substance abusing women to increase use of healthcare services or their adherence to a prescribed treatment regimen	• Outreach and prescreening of target population accomplished through existing agency efforts; characteristics of target population has shifted over time • Program actively links women to care both inside and outside PROTOTYPES continuum through active case management and referrals • Substance abusing women encouraged to enter treatment through linked PROTOTYPES programs; HIV-positive clients of PROTOTYPES residential substance abuse treatment program encouraged to receive services from WomensLink	• Outreach activities tracked through existing evaluations of those projects (funded by other sources) • Service linkages of WomensLink clients measured by Daily Services Form, Referral Form, chart review, follow-up interviews • Linkages to PROTOTYPES residential substance abuse treatment program identified through WomensLink program evaluation data, as well as separately maintained data systems at the residential program; allows monitoring of progress and outcomes of those women in that program	• 6,052 women in the hardest hit communities in Los Angeles received outreach and were screened for potential admission to WomensLink • 2,955 women who passed the pre-screening assessment were administered an individualized risk assessment • 404 women were enrolled in services • 250 women were linked via referrals to appropriate services • 393 women received case management • 305 of the women had at least one child under the age of 18; of those women, 285 received services related to their children
Goal 2: To change risk behaviors and prevent further HIV transmission by providing HIV/AIDS risk and transmission reduction counseling, HIV/AIDS antibody pre- and post-test counseling and peer counseling for those who test positive and negative for HIV antibody	• Program focuses on secondary prevention issues for women already identified as living with HIV through counseling, case management, support groups	• HIV prevention/intervention services monitored through Daily Services Form, chart review, follow-up interviews	• 1178 women received pre-test counseling; of those, 389 returned for their results

176

Goal	Activities	Measurement	Outcomes
Goal 3: To increase compliance with medical treatment and enhance access to existing services, by providing outreach to high need women, counseling to insure adherence to tuberculosis and other treatment regimens, and case management	• Adherence to treatment recommendations has remained a major focus of the WomensLink program, although TB did not present as a significant health issue among the women • Compliance issues changed as state-of-the-art medical care changed (i.e., introduction of combination therapy, HAART, viral load testing) • Different recommendations for pregnant women emerged during the project period, which also affected clinical management and adherence • Compliance issues among substance abusers has become a complicated clinical management issue; evolving medical education for staff and clients	• Direct services recorded on Daily Services Form, including those received from the Physician Assistant • Referrals to medical care and other services recorded on Referral Form • Adherence monitored through follow-up interviews, chart review, SF-21 Health-Related Quality of Life measure	• 394 of the 404 women received counseling and case management focused on medical treatment issues • 88 women referred to medical services or received services from the in-house physician assistant
Goal 4: To improve the quality of life for those individuals affected by and living with HIV/AIDS. The case manager will work with a woman throughout the entire continuum of services so as to insure that she receives all needed services in a coordinated, cost-effective, individually-appropriate way and that gaps and seams between services do not occur. The case manager will also help the woman learn to link with collateral community services. The buddy-sister and peer counseling programs will also help insure tight linkage	• The entire program is designed to maximize quality of life for clients • Case management has remained a cornerstone of the WomensLink model; case managers work with clients to address barriers to care • Individual and group therapy, health education, psychiatric consults, social events provide various methods designed to enhance quality of life • Peer counseling is funded through other sources, former clients have been hired as staff, internship opportunities; buddy-sister program did not catch on and was discontinued	• Case management services measured using Daily Services Form and Referral Form • Reduction of barriers measured using Barriers Form • Initial client needs measured using Needs Form • Quality of life measured using SF-21 Health-Related Quality of Life Form • Psychological distress measured using a short form of the Center for Epidemiological Studies Depression Scale • Staff observations of client status monitored through use of an Observations Form • Follow-up interviews used to examine long-term outcomes	• Clinical issues for 317 women were discussed by the treatment team in quarterly case conferences • Each woman had the same case manager throughout the course of her program involvement

and 4.2 percent women of other ethnic-racial backgrounds. The average age of the WomensLink clients is 35.9 years (standard deviation = 8.6 years), with clients ranging from 17 to 68 years of age. The women are from the poorest communities in Los Angeles, with 50.9 percent of the women living in precarious housing or being homeless. The majority of the women (91.0 percent) have a history of substance abuse. Most of the women (75.4 percent) have at least one child under the age of 18, many of whom are also living with HIV/AIDS.

Demonstration of Project Goals

Table 2 shows how the cumulative data inform the overall progress of the program in meeting its stated goals. As can be seen from the data summarized in Table 2, PROTOTYPES has provided outreach to more than 6,000 women in high-need communities and offered detailed risk assessments and referrals. The women seen by the outreach workers were provided the opportunity for HIV antibody testing, and if HIV-positive, were encouraged to enroll in WomensLink. Over the course of the project period, 404 women living with HIV/AIDS were enrolled in the program. Table 2 shows the number of women who received various services from WomensLink over the course of the project, including case management, substance abuse treatment, linkages to primary care, and other needed services.

Demonstration of Selected Project Outcomes

As discussed earlier, another major focus of this paper is to illustrate how outcomes can be evaluated in a community-based drop-in center where services are self-selected by the participants. The program has sought to reduce barriers to care for women with HIV/AIDS and consequently improve their health and psychosocial functioning. To demonstrate these outcomes, we implemented the "sweeps" methodology described above. The following summarizes the results of two repeated measures analyses of variance that address longitudinal change with respect to reduction of barriers to care and psychological distress. In each of these ANOVA models, two between-subjects design factors were included: (1) the number of days between the two administrations of the outcome measure (dichotomized as 365 days or less and more than 365 days between the two administrations), and (2) the relative service utilization rate per month (classified as participating in the program 2 days or fewer per month, 3-4 days per month, or at least 4 days per month). Each model also includes as a covariate the number of days from the woman's first service encounter to the earliest administration of the outcome measure. Table 3 summarizes the results of these two repeated measures ANOVAs. All significance levels are for one-tailed tests unless otherwise noted.

TABLE 3. Repeated Measures Analysis of Variance with Respect to Barriers to Care and Psychological Distress

Time of administration	Time between administrations	Service utilization rate	Perceived Barriers to Care — Observed N	Observed Mean	Observed Std. Dev.	Estimated[a] Mean	Estimated[a] Std. Error	Psychological Distress — Observed N	Observed Mean	Observed Std. Dev.	Estimated[a] Mean	Estimated[a] Std. Error
Earliest	≤ 365 days	≤ 2 days per month	13	4.53	2.96	4.39	.92	17	10.94	1.07	11.08	1.58
		3-4 days per month	14	5.29	2.85	5.53	.90	23	9.74	6.08	9.83	1.36
		≥ 4 days per month	17	5.24	3.67	5.16	.80	8	12.88	7.77	13.44	2.32
		Total	44	5.05	3.17	2.03	.50	48	10.69	6.68	11.45	1.04
	> 365 days	≤ 2 days per month	16	4.91	3.59	4.92	.83	21	10.24	7.38	9.96	1.43
		3-4 days per month	23	5.04	3.73	4.84	.69	26	12.42	5.54	12.46	1.28
		≥ 4 days per month	14	5.00	3.40	5.23	.92	27	11.78	6.88	12.03	1.26
		Total	53	4.99	3.53	5.00	.48	74	11.57	6.56	11.48	.76
	Total	≤ 2 days per month	29	4.74	3.27	4.66	.62	38	10.55	7.15	10.52	1.06
		3-4 days per month	37	5.14	3.38	5.19	.57	49	11.16	5.89	11.14	.93
		≥ 4 days per month	31	5.13	3.50	5.20	.61	35	12.03	6.99	12.73	1.32
		Total	97	5.02	3.36	5.01	.35	122	11.22	6.59	11.47	.64
Most recent	≤ 365 days	≤ 2 days per month	13	4.35	2.88	4.29	.90	17	9.53	6.02	9.55	1.53
		3-4 days per month	14	5.07	3.54	4.68	.88	23	9.78	7.38	9.59	1.33
		≥ 4 days per month	17	4.41	3.25	4.32	.79	8	16.13	4.73	16.05	2.25
		Total	44	4.60	3.18	4.43	.50	48	10.75	6.66	11.73	1.01
	> 365 days	≤ 2 days per month	16	4.22	3.57	4.25	.81	21	9.10	6.07	9.18	1.39
		3-4 days per month	23	3.74	3.20	3.86	.68	26	10.73	6.85	10.59	1.24
		≥ 4 days per month	14	3.89	4.17	4.49	.91	27	7.93	5.58	7.96	1.22
		Total	53	3.92	3.52	4.20	.47	74	9.24	6.22	9.24	.74
	Total	≤ 2 days per month	29	4.28	3.22	4.27	.61	38	9.29	5.97	9.36	1.03
		3-4 days per month	37	4.24	3.35	4.27	.56	49	10.29	7.04	10.09	.91
		≥ 4 days per month	31	4.18	3.63	4.41	.60	35	9.80	6.37	12.01	1.29
		Total	97	4.23	3.37	4.32	.34	122	9.84	6.50	10.48	.63

[a]Estimated marginal means accounting for the effect of the covariate, days from first service encounter to first outcome assessment.

Barriers to care. In this analysis, we compared the level of barriers reported at the earliest assessment to that at the woman's most recent assessment. A total of 97 women had data from more than one assessment of barriers to care, with the assessments being at least 30 days apart. In this model, the main effect for earliest versus most recent barriers assessment was statistically significant, $F(1,87) = 5.021$, $p < .05$. The mean barrier scores were 5.0 (s.d. = 3.4) at the earliest assessment and 4.2 (s.d. = 3.4) at the most recent assessment. When considering the effects of the covariate of days from initiating services to the baseline assessment of barriers, the interaction of the earliest versus most recent assessment and service utilization rate was statistically significant, $F(2,87) = 3.231$, $p < .05$. As can be seen in Table 3, barriers decreased the least for women with the lowest service utilization rates. The interaction of earliest versus most recent assessment by service utilization rate–not including the effect of the covariate–was not statistically significant, $(F(2,87) = .926$, $p = .200)$, nor was the interaction of earliest versus most recent assessment by days between assessments, $F(1,87) = .383$, $p = .269)$, or the interaction of earliest versus most recent assessment by service utilization rates by days between the assessments, $F(1,87) = .044$, $p = .478$. Including the effects of the covariate (time from initiating services to the baseline assessment of barriers), the main effect of earliest versus most recent assessment was non-significant, $F(1,87) = 2.432$, $p = .061$, as was the interaction of earliest versus most recent assessment by days between assessments, $F(1,87) = .650$, $p = .211$.

There were also some statistically significant between-group differences. The covariate of days from the initial service encounter to the first barriers assessment differentiated the women in this sample, $F(1,87) = 5.794$, $p < .05$, as did the interaction of service utilization rate by the covariate, $F(2,87) = 4.207$, $p < .05$. The remaining between-group factors were not statistically significant, including service utilization rate $(F(2,87) = .895$, $p = .206)$, days between assessments $(F(1,87) = .036$, $p = .424)$, the interaction of service utilization rate by days between assessments $(F(2,87) = .409$, $p = .333)$, and the interaction of days between assessments by the covariate $(F(1,87) = .641$, $p = .212)$.

Psychological distress. In this analysis we compared the level of psychological distress as measured by the CES-D at the earliest assessment to that obtained at the woman's most recent assessment. A total of 122 women had data from more than one CES-D administration, with the assessments being at least 30 days apart. In this model, the main effect for earliest versus most recent CES-D assessment was significant, at the .05 level, $F(1,112) = 2.699$. The mean CES-D score was 11.2 (s.d. = 6.6) at the earliest assessment and 9.8 (s.d. = 6.5) at the most recent assessment. There was also a significant effect for the interaction of the earliest versus most recent assessment and days between administrations, $F(1,112) = 4.061, p < .05$. As shown in Table 3, women with more than one year between their first and last CES-D assessments demonstrated a reduction in psychological distress, whereas those with less than one year between the assessments did not. In addition, the interaction of earliest versus most recent assessment by service utilization rate by days between assessments was significant, $F(2,112) = 2.378, p < .05$. As shown in Table 3, the greatest reduction in CES-D Scores was demonstrated by those women who participated at least weekly and who had at least a year between assessments. The interaction of earliest versus most recent assessment by service utilization rate did not reach statistical significance, $F(2,112) = 1.728, p = .091$.

Including the effect of the covariate of days from the initial service visit to the first CES-D administration, there was a statistically significant interaction of earliest versus most recent assessment by service utilization rate by the covariate, $F(2,112) = 5.421, p < .001$. The other interactions involving the covariate were not statistically significant, including the interaction of earliest versus most recent assessment by the covariate $(F(1,112) = .346, p = .278)$ and the interaction of earliest versus most recent assessment by days between assessments by the covariate $(F(1,112) = .310, p = .289)$.

In terms of between-group differences, the only statistically significant effect was for the interaction of service utilization rate and days between assessments, $F(2,112) = 2.904, p < .05$. The remaining between-group factors did not reach statistical significance, including service utilization rate $(F(2,112) = .404, p = .334)$, days between the assessments $(F(1,112) = 1.492, p = .112)$, the covariate of time from first service encounter to baseline distress assessment $(F(1,112) = .590, p = .222)$, the interaction of service utilization rate by the covariate $(F(2,112) = 1.452, p = .114)$, and the interaction of days between assessments by the covariate $(F(1,112) = .185, p = .334)$.

DISCUSSION

In this paper, we have shown how an evaluation can define progress towards program goals and objectives to illustrate the flow of clients through a conceptual model. In doing so, we can use the information about each of the goals to evaluate the program's ability to implement the model that was initially proposed. In the case of PROTOTYPES WomensLink, the program has successfully demonstrated the implementation of a continuum of care for women with HIV, from the initial community contact to engaging and retaining the woman in a gender-specific, culturally sensitive model of care. We have provided this information to illustrate the utility of program evaluation for community-based organizations providing services to women with HIV.

It is critical to take a flexible approach in designing and implementing evaluations of community-based services. Evaluating such programs requires attention to both programmatic concerns and evaluation considerations. It is important that community-based organizations have the opportunity to contribute to the body of knowledge about what constitutes effective HIV/AIDS services for women and their families. In the case of evaluating the Womens-Link model program, programmatic and evaluation concerns have been integrated from the program's inception. This integration continues to inform decision-making by program managers after five years of engaging and retaining women and their families in care. By ensuring that program and evaluation elements are planned and implemented in parallel, the evaluation can remain responsive to the needs of the women and to the service delivery model that evolves to meet those needs. For example, consider the incentives used to attract women to participate in follow-up evaluation interviews. The incentives were carefully chosen jointly by program and evaluation staff so that they would best meet the needs of the women. Vouchers were provided so that women could choose which necessities–whether food, clothing, or items for their family–they could obtain in stores located in their communities, thereby eliminating the need for transportation. In addition, providing the vouchers helped the women to work with program staff to develop life skills such as budgeting and planning how to use these community resources. In short, something that initially was seen as a method for increasing response rate for an evaluation procedure also was used as an opportunity to provide a programmatic intervention.

In focusing on "practical issues" in evaluating a community-based program for women living with HIV/AIDS, this article provides concrete exemplars of many of the theoretical issues addressed by Huba, Brown, Melchior, Hughes, and Panter (this volume). Most of these issues are likely to be relevant for evaluating other similar community-based services, and are not specific to evaluating a program for women with HIV/AIDS. Yet the model of evaluation employed here, using many tenets of empowerment evaluation (e.g., Fetterman, 1994; Smith, 1998) evolved into one that reflected the cultural competence and woman-centered aspects (such as those related to children, caregiver roles, and reproductive issues; e.g., Crystal & Sambamoorthi, 1996) of the program.

Issues of cultural competence are critical in designing programs that maximize outcomes for various ethnic and cultural groups. We consider one of the biggest successes of the WomensLink program to be the fact that evaluation results did not differ by racial-ethnic group (see Brown, Melchior, Hughes, & Huba, 1999). Being able to evaluate whether critical program outcomes such as engagement and retention in various services and long-term changes in access to care, psychosocial adjustment, and overall health and functioning differ across key groups targeted by the program is important to demonstrate that the program is equally relevant for all its participants. In addition, developing evaluation measures or translating existing measures into Spanish in the local dialect by translators knowledgeable in healthcare issues helped to make these measures accessible to the substantial number of Spanish-speaking clients of the program–both those who are monolingual, as well as those who are bilingual but are more comfortable responding to questions in their native language. By continually coordinating and linking program and evaluation, it is possible to maximize the cultural relevance and appropriateness of program and evaluation procedures in a multicultural environment.

In conclusion, the WomensLink program has demonstrated how program and evaluation staff can collaborate to produce an evaluation that is useful for clinical, administrative, and evaluation purposes. It is critical to begin this collaboration as early as possible, ideally at the time of the initial program development. By thoroughly integrating program and evaluation issues every step of the way, the best possible data can be obtained to replicate the model program so that care for all women with HIV can be made as relevant and accessible as possible.

REFERENCES

Bozzette, S. A., Hays, R. D., Wu, A. W., Berry, S. H., & Kanouse, D. (1995). Derivation and psychometric properties of a brief health-related quality of life instrument for HIV disease. *Journal of Acquired Immunodeficiency Syndromes and Retrovirology, 8,* 253-265.

Brown, V. B., Hughes, A., Melchior, L. A., & Huba, G. J. (1998, November). *Design of a settlement house model program for women with HIV/AIDS.* Presented at the annual meetings of the American Public Health Association, Washington, DC.

Brown, V. B., Melchior, L. A., Hughes, C., & Huba, G. J. (2000). Enhancing HIV treatment access and outcomes for women of color. Under review.

Campbell, C. (1999). *Women, Families, & HIV/AIDS: A Sociological Perspective on the Epidemic in America.* New York: Cambridge University Press.

Centers for Disease Control and Prevention (1999). *HIV/AIDS Surveillance Report, 11* (1), 1-44.

Crystal, S., & Sambamoorthi, U. (1996). Care needs and access to care among women living with HIV. In L. Sherr, C. Hankins, & L. Bennett (Eds.), *AIDS as a Gender Issue.* Bristol, PA: Taylor & Francis.

Fetterman, D. M. (1994). Steps of empowerment evaluation: From California to Cape Town. *Evaluation & Program Planning, 17* (3), Special Feature, 305-313.

Huba, G. J. & Melchior, L. A. (1996, August). Technical and practical design issues in cross-site HIV service evaluations. In G. Huba (Chair), *Cross-site evaluations of HIV services: Technical issues and experiences.* Presented at the American Psychological Association Meeting, Toronto.

Huba, G. J., & Melchior, L. A. (1994). *Evaluation of the Effects of Ryan White Title I Funding on Services for HIV-Infected Drug Abusers: Summary Report & Execu-*

tive Summary for Year 1: Baseline. US Dept. of Health and Human Services Pub No. HRSA-RD-SP-94-8. A joint project of the Health Resources and Services Administration, the National Institute on Drug Abuse, and the Consortium on Drug Abuse and HIV Services Access.

Huba, G. J., Brown, V. B., Melchior, L. A., Hughes, C., & Panter, A. T. (2000). Conceptual issues in implementing and using evaluation in the "real world" setting of a community-based organization for HIV/AIDS services. *Drugs & Society, 16* (1/2), 31-54.

Huba, G. J., Melchior, L. A., Panter, A. T., Brown, V. B., & Larson, T. A. (2000). A national program of AIDS care projects and their cross-cutting evaluation: The HRSA SPNS Cooperative Agreements. *Drugs & Society, 16* (1/2), 5-29.

Huba, G. J., Melchior, L. A., Staff of The Measurement Group, and the HRSA SPNS Cooperative Agreement Projects (1995). *Module 26: Current Psychological Distress Form.* Available: www.TheMeasurementGroup.com/.

Los Angeles County Department of Health Services, HIV Epidemiology Program. (1999, July). *Advanced HIV Disease (AIDS) Surveillance Summary*, 1-27.

Melchior, L. A., Huba, G. J., Brown, V. B., & Reback, C. J. (1993). A short depression index for women. *Educational and Psychological Measurement, 53* (4), 1117-1125.

Raveis, V. H., Siegel, K., & Gorey, E. (1998). Factors associated with HIV-infected women's delay in seeking medical care. *AIDS Care, 10* (5), 549-562.

Rosen, D., & Blank, W. (1992). Women and HIV. In H. Land (Ed.), *AIDS: A complete guide to psychosocial intervention.* pp. 141-151. Milwaukee, WI: Family Service America, 300 pages.

Russell, J. M., & Smith, K. (1998). HIV infected women and women's services. *Healthcare for Women International, 19* (2), 131-139.

Siegel, K., Karus, D., & Raveis, V. H. (1997). Testing and treatment behavior of HIV-infected women: White, African-American, Puerto Rican comparisons. *AIDS Care, 9* (3), 297-309.

Smith, M. K. (1998). Empowerment evaluation: Theoretical and methodological considerations. *Evaluation & Program Planning, 21* (3), 255-261.

Stober, D. R., Schwartz, J. A. J., McDaniel, J. S., & Abrams, R. F. (1997). Depression and HIV disease: Prevalence, correlates, and treatment. *Psychiatric Annals, 27* (5), 372-377.

Weissman, G., & Brown, V. B. (1996). Drug-using women and HIV: Access to care and treatment issues. In A. O'Leary, L. S. Jemmott et al. (Eds.), *Women and AIDS: Coping and care*, pp. 109-121. New York: Plenum.

Weissman, G., Melchior, L., Huba, G., Altice, F., Booth, R., Cottler, L., Genser, S., Jones, A., McCarthy, S., Needle, R., & Smereck, G. (1995). Women living with substance abuse and HIV disease: Medical care access issues. *Journal of the American Medical Women's Association, 50* (3-4), 115-120.

Weissman, G., Melchior, L., Huba, G., Smereck, G., Needle, R., McCarthy, S., Jones, A., Genser, S., Cottler, L., Booth, R., & Altice, F. (1995). Women living with drug abuse and HIV disease: Drug treatment access and secondary prevention issues. *Journal of Psychoactive Drugs, 27* (4), 401-412.

Substance Abuse
and Health Services Utilization
Among Women
in a Comprehensive HIV Program

Karen L. Meredith, MPH, RN, CHES
Donna B. Jeffe, PhD
Victoria J. Fraser, MD
Linda M. Mundy, MD

SUMMARY. Substance abuse history and treatment needs were assessed in 308 women at a comprehensive HIV program in St. Louis. We found that 229 (74%) women had a history of substance abuse and 38 (12%) had a history of injection drug use. Only 25 (44%) of 57 women

Karen L. Meredith and Linda M. Mundy are affiliated with the Division of Infectious Diseases, Department of Internal Medicine, Washington University School of Medicine, St. Louis, MO, and the Helena Hatch Special Care Center, St. Louis, MO. Donna B. Jeffe is affiliated with the Division of Health Behavior Research, Departments of Internal Medicine and Pediatrics, Washington University School of Medicine, St. Louis, MO. Victoria J. Fraser is affiliated with the Division of Infectious Diseases, Department of Internal Medicine, Washington University School of Medicine.

Address correspondence to: Linda M. Mundy, MD, Washington University School of Medicine, Campus Box 8051, 660 South Euclid Avenue, St. Louis, MO 63110 (E-mail: lmundy@imgate.wustl.edu).

This work was supported in part by the Health Resources and Services Administration (HRSA), HIV/AIDS Bureau (HAB), Special Projects of National Significance (SPNS) Grant No. 5 U90 HA 00042-05. This publication's contents are solely the responsibility of the authors and do not necessarily represent the official view of the funding agency.

[Haworth co-indexing entry note]: "Substance Abuse and Health Services Utilization Among Women in a Comprehensive HIV Program." Meredith, Karen L. et al. Co-published simultaneously in *Drugs & Society* (The Haworth Press, Inc.) Vol. 16, No. 1/2, 2000, pp. 185-201; and: *Evaluating HIV/AIDS Treatment Programs: Innovative Methods and Findings* (ed: G. J. Huba et al.) The Haworth Press, Inc., 2000, pp. 185-201. Single or multiple copies of this article are available for a fee from The Haworth Document Delivery Service [1-800-342-9678, 9:00 a.m. - 5:00 p.m. (EST). E-mail address: getinfo@haworthpressinc.com].

requiring substance abuse treatment at enrollment had received treatment. Adherence with quarterly medical follow-up was associated with highly active antiretroviral therapy (HAART) prescription in 1997 and 1998, but not with need for substance abuse treatment. However, women needing substance abuse treatment were less likely to have been prescribed HAART in 1998. We recommend that providers of medical services to women with HIV conduct formal assessments of substance abuse behaviors among their patients and ensure that treatment needs are adequately addressed within the framework of care. Further examination of the use of HAART in women who are active substance abusers is needed. *[Article copies available for a fee from The Haworth Document Delivery Service: 1-800-342-9678. E-mail address: <getinfo@haworthpress inc.com> Website: <http://www.HaworthPress.com>]*

KEYWORDS. Substance abuse, HIV, women, evaluation, comprehensive care

INTRODUCTION

Women, especially those who are poor and/or of ethnic minorities, comprise the fastest growing number of incident cases of HIV in the United States (Centers for Disease Control and Prevention, 1997). The primary risk factor for HIV among women has changed over the past decade from injecting drug use (IDU) to heterosexual transmission (Weissman, Melchior, Huba, Altice, Booth, Cottler, Genser, Jones, McCarthy, Needle, & Smereck, 1995). However, substance abuse continues to be a major contributor to HIV infection among women, particularly through unprotected heterosexual contact with an HIV-infected IDU partner, sex for drug barter activities and other high-risk behaviors facilitated by drug-induced exhilaration or disinhibition (Weissman, Melchior, Huba, Altice, Booth, Cottler, Genser, Jones, McCarthy, Needle, & Smereck, 1995). Regardless of the actual source of HIV transmission, substance abuse is a major issue for many women with HIV in this country, with the majority reported to be active or recovering drug users (Weissman, Melchior, Huba, Altice, Booth, Cottler, Genser, Jones, McCarthy, Needle, & Smereck, 1995). Substance abuse has also been associated with increased unemployment, poverty, and comorbidity such as mental illness (Weissman, Melchior, Huba, Altice, Booth, Cottler, Genser, Jones, McCarthy, Needle, & Smereck, 1995). Limited access to HIV treatment has been noted among drug-dependent populations, either due to delayed clinical diagnosis, barriers to service delivery, or behavioral factors (Barbour, 1998; Flanigan, Merriman, Dickinson, Fiore, Tashima, Mitty et al., 1998; Hirschhorn, Quinones, Goldin, & Metras, 1998; Weissman, Melchior, Huba, Altice, Booth, Cottler, Genser, Jones, McCarthy, Needle, & Smereck, 1995). Many women with co-occurring substance abuse and HIV are underrepresented in HIV care programs. Among 140 women attending an HIV/AIDS prenatal clinic between 1990 and 1993, 40-50% were current substance abusers by self-report or toxicology screening (Bardequez, Wesley, Grandchamp, Gaines, & Newsome, 1995). A 1996 report of 40 women seeking care at a Chicago women's HIV clinic showed that 53% were actively using "street" drugs and 48% had a history of IDU (Nelson, Ferrando, Stanislawski & Garcia, 1996).

Active substance abuse was not initially considered a common behavior among enrollees at this Midwest site because: (1) few women reported active substance abuse to healthcare staff, (2) heterosexual transmission was identified as the primary route of HIV transmission, and (3) the prevalence of IDU is relatively low in this metropolitan area. As enrollment increased from 25 patients in 1995 to over 300 in 1998, our staff became increasingly cognizant of patients with drug use behaviors who had eluded medical diagnoses and treatment. We therefore felt it was critical to evaluate the prevalence of substance use and treatment needs among women receiving care at our site and to identify improved methods for evaluating substance abuse among women in this HIV comprehensive care program. The purpose of this study was to evaluate the substance abuse history and treatment needs among a cohort of women enrolled at a comprehensive HIV-care program in St. Louis, Missouri.

METHODS

The Helena Hatch Special Care Center (HHSCC) is a comprehensive HIV program for women based at Washington University School of Medicine in St. Louis, Missouri. The program is funded by a five-year Special Projects of National Significance (SPNS) program grant from the Health Resources and Services Administration. HHSCC provides a full-range of medical and psychosocial services in a one-stop-shop environment, in conjunction with a wide range of evaluation activities. For this study, data on substance use and alcohol abuse were assessed for 308 women enrolled at the HHSCC between January 1, 1995 and August 1, 1998.

Demographic data (age at enrollment and time of the study, residence at enrollment, and education) and medical data (date of HIV diagnosis and CD4 cell counts) were obtained from the HHSCC clinical database. Nadir CD4 cell count was defined as the lowest CD4 count ever measured for each patient. Substance abuse data were aggregated from several sources including self-report surveys, case notes of case managers, and the medical records (reflecting random clinician notes and drug testing reports). This information was collected at program enrollment for each patient and then updated throughout the continuum of patient care by medical and social support staff. Many of the women completed annual substance abuse surveys (Module 24, *Brief Substance Abuse History Form*; Huba, Melchior, Staff of The Measurement Group, and the HRSA SPNS Program Cooperative Agreement Projects, 1997a) in 1996 ($n = 70$), in 1997 ($n = 124$), and in 1998 ($n = 169$) as part of our ongoing program evaluation. Survey responses identified a history of substance abuse for alcohol and various illicit drugs (marijuana, cocaine and/or crack, heroin, amphetamines, or non-physician-prescribed medications) and whether or not there was a history of IDU. Self-reported underage drinking (due to its illegal nature), injecting alcohol, binge drinking or being recommended for or receiving alcohol-related treatment defined alcohol abuse. From the survey data, we dichotomized the age at which respondents first began drinking alcohol to group those drinking before they were 21 and those who reported drinking at or after the age of 21. By default, women with unknown age for initiation of alcohol consumption were grouped in the over-21 category. Substance abuse data had been coded as current, ever, never, or unknown in each of the various sources of data. Current substance abuse was inadequately measured because multiple sources of information were used to collect these data over time. Therefore, having a history of substance abuse included records of either past or current abuse of each specific substance, and unknown substance abuse included never having used and unknown use of each substance.

From case notes, data were obtained regarding need for substance abuse treatment. As part of regular care, case managers screened for this need using the following questions: "Has anyone described you as having a problem with this substance? Has a friend or doctor asked you to go to rehabilitation for using this substance? Have you ever passed out or done something you didn't want to because of using this substance?" Women's receipt of inpatient or outpatient substance abuse treatment also was recorded.

Utilization of health services utilization in 1997 was based on number of medical (clinic) visits per quarter and number of nursing/social work-case management interventions. Numbers of clinic visits for medical care were obtained from the medical records. Optimal medical care, especially for women taking highly active antiretroviral therapy (HAART), required at least one clinic visit every three months to monitor plasma HIV RNA levels and CD4 cell counts (Carpenter, Fischl, Hammer et al., 1998; Report of the NIH Panel, 1998). Medical care was categorized as a proportion of time enrolled in 1997 for which women had clinic visits: 0 = having no visits during any quarter enrolled in 1997; 1 = having visits less than half the time enrolled; 2 = having visits during only half the time enrolled; 3 = having visits more than half the time enrolled; 4 = having at least one clinic visit during all quarters enrolled at HHSCC in 1997 (optimal). Using this graded coding scheme, we could take into consideration time in which women were either not enrolled at HHSCC or deceased.

We measured nursing/case management time and effort using the Module

2B, *Intervention-Services Form* (Huba, Melchior, Staff of The Measurement Group, & the HRSA SPNS Program Cooperative Agreement Projects, 1997b). The Module 2B data were summarized as the number of individual encounters with a nurse/nurse practitioner or with a case manager/social worker and total time (in minutes) per encounter. Categories of encounters included patient education, HIV prevention/intervention, mental health, substance abuse, and case management/advocacy. In addition, "other" services included activities at HHSCC, being accompanied to the hospital, family planning, information and referral, recreation, and transportation. Only services provided on an individual basis (not in-group settings) were included in the summary data of Module 2B.

Data Analysis

Statistical tests were conducted using SPSS 8.0.2. Two-tailed tests were considered statistically significant at $p < .05$. Chi-square tests of significance were used to measure associations among use of each of the various substances, whether or not women needed or received treatment for substance abuse, race (Caucasian, African American, and Hispanic), and residence at enrollment (in the City of St. Louis vs. all other cities combined). The significance of Fisher's exact tests are reported for all 2×2 tests of the associations among substance abuse variables (e.g., among the various pairs of substances). Age at enrollment, level of education (i.e., number of years of formal schooling), multiple substance use, clinic visits, and the number and minutes of nurse/social work-case management interventions were treated as continuous variables. Analyses of variance tested the significance of the differences in these variables by each of the substance abuse variables, underage drinking, race, and residence at enrollment.

Pearson correlations assessed the relationships among multiple illicit drug use, optimal care, the number of nurse/social work-case management interventions, and amount of time provided during nurse/social work-case management interventions. Multiple linear regression assessed the independent predictors of optimal medical care, the number of nurse/social work-case management interventions, and time allocations per intervention. Multiple logistic regression identified independent predictors of use of HAART in 1997 and 1998 and women's need for substance abuse treatment using the likelihood-ratio criteria for stepwise variable entry (.05) and removal (.10).

RESULTS

Of 308 women who were enrolled at HHSCC as of August 1, 1998, 229 (74.4%) resided in the metropolitan St. Louis area at enrollment, the majority of whom resided in the City of St. Louis at enrollment ($n = 169$; 54.9%)

(Figure 1). Of the 277 (90%) women still living on August 1, 1998, 202 (72.9%) resided in the St. Louis surveillance area, accounting for 77.1% of all 262 women over the age of 12 living with HIV in the St. Louis metropolitan surveillance area (G. Harvey, personal communication, December 23, 1998). The median age at enrollment was 27.0 years, and among the women still living, the median age was 29.0 years. The majority of women were African American (76.6%), 22.1% were Caucasian, and 1.3% were Hispanic or Asian/Pacific Islander. One hundred ninety-one of the 299 women with education data (63.9%) had at least completed high school. The mean (standard deviation) number of years of schooling was 11.68 ± 1.82). There was no significant relationship observed between education and age at enrollment. The initial median CD4 cell count at enrollment for 294 women with available CD4 data was 365 cells/mm^3 (range 1 to 1730 cells/mm^3). For 262 women still alive and reporting a date of HIV diagnosis, the median number of years living with HIV disease was 3 years (range 0-13 years). Overall, nearly three-quarters (74.4%) of the sample reported some substance abuse history. Only four women were known to abuse prescription painkillers or barbiturates that were not prescribed by a physician; therefore, abuse of these drugs was not further analyzed.

Substance abuse. As shown in Table 1, intercorrelations of the numbers and percentages of women abusing various pairs of substances revealed that use of one substance was significantly associated with use of other substances.

Associations between substance abuse, residence, age at enrollment, and education. Women who resided in the city of St. Louis at enrollment were more likely to have ever smoked tobacco (114/169 [67.5%] vs. 75/139 [54.0%]; $p = .019$), abused alcohol (109/169 [64.5%] vs. 69/139 [49.6%]; $p = .011$), smoked marijuana (108/169 [63.9%] vs. 72/139 [51.8%]; $p = .037$), and used cocaine/crack (62/169 [36.7%] vs. 34/139 [24.5%]; $p = .026$) compared to women living in other parts in Missouri and Illinois. Women with a history of marijuana use were younger at enrollment compared to women whose history of marijuana use was unknown (mean age 28 vs. 30; $p = .044$). Women with a history of smoking tobacco (mean age 28 vs. 30; $p = .044$), using cocaine/crack (mean age 32 vs. 27; $p < .001$), heroin (mean age 34 vs. 29; $p = .002$), IDU (mean age 36 vs. 28; $p < .001$), and amphetamines (mean age 34 vs. 29; $p = .008$) were significantly older at enrollment compared to women with an unknown history for use of these substances. In addition, women with a history of cocaine/crack use tended to have fewer years of formal schooling compared to women whose history of cocaine/crack use was unknown (mean years of schooling 11 vs. 12; $p = .036$).

Underage drinking. Of 144 women reporting an age for first drinking alcohol, 123 (85.4%) reported consuming alcohol before the age of 21. Underage drinking was associated with use of marijuana (110/123 [89.4%] vs.

FIGURE 1. Distribution of Women Enrolled at HHSCC by County

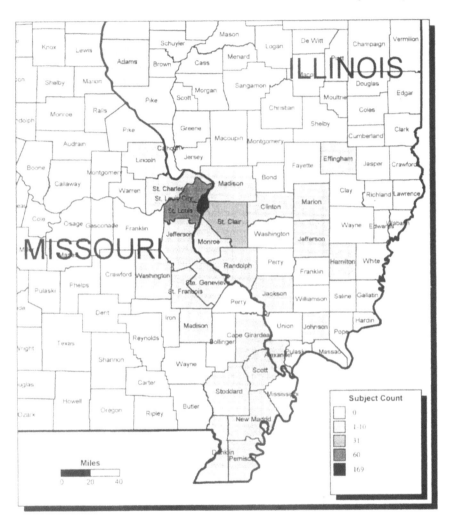

70/185 [37.8%]; *p* < .001) and amphetamines (18/123 [14.6%] vs. 5/185 [2.7%]; *p* < .001), but was not significantly associated with education or with use of tobacco, cocaine/crack, heroin, IDU, or needle sharing.

Use of multiple drugs. The majority (*n* = 171, 84.6%) reported a history of abuse of two or more substances including alcohol. Forty-nine women reported a history of using only one substance, with 22 reporting alcohol abuse, 21 reporting marijuana use, and 6 reporting cocaine/crack use. Excluding

TABLE 1. Associations of Known History of Substance Abuse(s) Among Women with HIV

	n	Tobacco	Alcohol	Marijuana	Cocaine/Crack	Heroin	IDU	Amphetamines
Tobacco	189	—						
Alcohol	178	123 (69.1)****	—					
Marijuana	180	127 (70.6)****	144 (80.0)****	—				
Cocaine/Crack	96	82 (85.4)****	77 (80.2)****	79 (82.3)****	—			
Heroin	29	27 (93.1)****	26 (89.7)****	25 (86.2)****	23 (79.3)****	—		
IDU	38	34 (89.5)****	31 (81.6)****	29 (76.3)****	24 (63.2)****	20 (52.6)****	—	
Amphetamines	23	18 (78.3)	21 (91.3)****	23(100.0)****	15 (65.2)****	8 (34.8)****	9 (39.1)****	—
Needed Treatment	57	51 (89.5)****	48 (84.2)****	47 (82.5)****	46 (80.7)****	11 (19.3)**	13 (22.8)*	5 (8.8)
Received Inpatient	20	19 (95.0)****	18 (90.0)***	17 (85.0)*	20 (100.0)****	5 (25.0)*	6 (30.0)*	1 (5.0)
Received Outpatient	25	22 (88.0)***	22 (88.0)****	22 (88.0)****	24 (96.0)****	6 (24.0)*	7 (28.0)*	3 (12.0)

Notes.
$N = 308$. Values in parentheses are percentages of n.
IDU = Injecting Drug Use.
Tests of significance are two-tailed Fisher's exact.
*$p < .05$. **$p < .01$. ***$p < .005$. ****$p < .001$

192

alcohol abuse, 94 (30.5%) reported use of two or more illicit substances. There was no correlation between the number of years of schooling and use of multiple drugs ($r = -.086; p = .139$). Women living in the city of St. Louis reported using a greater number of substances compared to women living in other areas (mean 1.85 vs. 1.42; $p = .005$). In addition, women with a history of smoking tobacco used greater numbers of substances compared to non-tobacco smokers (mean 2.01 vs. 1.09; $p < .001$). Women with a history of alcohol abuse used a greater number of illicit substances compared to women whose abuse of alcohol was unknown (mean 1.52 vs. 0.48; $p < .001$). Underage drinking also was associated with use of greater numbers of illicit substances compared to women whose drinking age was unknown (mean 1.55 vs. 0.76; $p < .001$).

Needing or receiving treatment for substance abuse. The associations between need for and receipt of substance abuse treatment and use of each of the various substances are shown in Table 1. Fifty-seven (18.5%) women were reported to be in need of substance abuse treatment while enrolled at HHSCC. Women living in the city of St. Louis at enrollment (43/169 [25.4%] vs. 14/139 [10.1%]; $p = .001$) were more likely to have needed substance abuse treatment compared to women living outside the city. Women needing substance abuse treatment had used a greater number of illicit substances on average compared to women who were not identified as needing treatment (1.91 vs. 0.89; $p < .001$). Twenty-five (8.1%) women were known to have received outpatient treatment for substance abuse, representing 43.9% of those 57 women in need of treatment. Of these 25 women, 16 (64.0%) reported underage drinking compared to 107 of 283 (37.8%) women whose outpatient treatment history was unknown ($p = .017$).

Impact of substance abuse on health services utilization. To assess the impact of substance abuse on utilization of clinical resources, we analyzed associations between the substance abuse variables and adherence with quarterly medical visits, number of nurse/social work-case management interventions, time allocations per intervention, and being prescribed HAART in 1997 and 1998. These analyses were conducted on the subset ($n = 202$) for whom we had complete data for 1997 clinic visits (to compute optimal medical care; $n = 208$) and services (Module 2B; $n = 308$), for prescribed use of antiretroviral therapy in 1997 and 1998 ($n = 296$), and for substance abuse ($n = 308$). This subset of 202 women was more likely to have been taking HAART in 1997 (20.8% vs. 2.1%; $p < .001$) and in 1998 (36.1% vs. 22.3%; $p = .022$) and to have been younger at enrollment (mean age 28 vs. 32 years; $p < .001$) compared to the 106 women without complete data. These two groups of women did not differ in terms of education, length of time since being diagnosed with HIV, initial CD4 cell counts at enrollment, or minimum CD4 counts.

Descriptive statistics of clinic visits and staff interventions. Adherence with medical care scores ranged from zero to four. For the entire 1997 period of enrollment at HHSCC, 77 of 202 (38.1%) women presented for optimal medical care (at least one clinic visit per quarter), 50 women (24.8%) had clinic visits more than half the time they were enrolled, 39 women (19.3%) had clinic visits half the time they were enrolled, 23 (11.4%) had clinic visits less than half the time they were enrolled, and 13 women (6.4%) had no clinic visits during the period they were enrolled in 1997. The mean score for annual clinic visits was 2.8, and the median was 3.0. Only 42 women (20.8%) were prescribed HAART in 1997, compared to 73 women (36.1%) by July 1998.

There were a total of 4,714 reports of nurse/social work-case management interventions provided to individual women at HHSCC in 1997. Of these only 12 were for substance abuse, of which all were provided by a case manager or social worker to six of 202 (3.0%) women. The time range for these interventions ranged from 10 to 162 minutes. Half of the total interventions provided (2,381) were for case management/advocacy and 172 services were provided for HIV prevention/intervention. In addition, 462 mental health services and 1,687 "other" services were provided.

Bivariate analyses. In bivariate correlations using the subset of 202 women, adherence with quarterly medical clinic visits positively correlated with the number of interventions by a nurse/nurse practitioner ($r = .287, p < .001$) and the number of minutes in services with a nurse/nurse practitioner ($r = .326, p < .001$). Number of interventions and time with a case manager or social worker were not significantly related to adherence with quarterly medical visits. There was a significant association between multiple illicit drug use history with the number of minutes with a nurse/nurse practitioner ($r = .196, p = .005$) and the number of interventions with a nurse/nurse practitioner ($r = .184, p = .009$) and with a case manager/social worker ($r = .165, p = .020$). In addition, women with a history of cocaine/crack use were significantly less likely to be prescribed HAART in 1998 compared to women whose history of cocaine/crack use was unknown (chi-square tests 23.3% vs. 76.7%; $p = .043$). Women in need of substance abuse treatment also were less likely to be prescribed HAART in 1997 (7.3% vs. 24.2%; $p = .017$) and in 1998 (9.8% vs. 42.9%; $p < .001$) compared to women whose needs for treatment were unknown.

Multivariate analyses. Stepwise multiple linear regression analyses identified significant predictors of optimal medical visits and staff interventions among the demographic data, substance abuse variables, HAART prescription in 1997, and each of the other service and medical care variables (see Table 2). History of some substance abuse correlated significantly with quarterly medical visits and three of the four nurse/social work-case management intervention variables. But in each case, the substance abuse variables accounted for only a small proportion of the variance of each of the dependent variables.

TABLE 2. Multiple Linear Recessions of Optimal Medical Visits and Staff Interventions

Variables in order of entry	Total R^2 at entry	Standardized Coefficients (Final Beta)	t	p
Interventions (No.)				
Nurse/nurse practitioner (minutes)	.887	.942	39.67	< .001
Case manager/social worker (minutes)	.653	.764	18.55	< .001
Alcohol abuse history	.667	.091	2.18	.030
Resided in city of St. Louis at enrollment	.676	.096	2.35	.020
Heroin abuse history	.684	.099	2.41	.017
Education	.691	.083	2.09	.038
Duration of Nurse/Nurse Practitioner Interventions				
Nurse/nurse practitioner (interventions)	.887	.901	36.40	< .001
Case manager/social worker (minutes)	.892	.078	3.25	.001
Quarterly medical visits	.895	.057	2.39	.018
Amphetamine use history	.898	.047	2.05	.041
Duration of Case Management/Social Work Interventions				
Case manager/social worker (interventions)	.653	.772	18.41	< .001
Nurse/nurse practitioner (minutes)	.664	− .154	3.51	.001
Prescribed HAART in 1997	.675	− .105	− 2.51	.013
Injecting drug use history	.683	− .087	− 2.15	.033
Quarterly Medical Visits in 1997				
Prescribed HAART in 1997	.069	.252	3.96	< .001
Years with known HIV infection	.130	− .250	− 3.95	< .001
Alcohol abuse history	.179	.220	3.48	.001
Nurse/nurse practitioner (minutes)	.211	.178	2.80	.006

Note. N = 202 (subset of respondents with complete data).

Logistic regression identified significant independent predictors of needing substance abuse treatment and of use of HAART in 1997 and 1998 from among the substance abuse variables, demographic data, and clinic visits, and each of the staff interventions (Table 3). Significant independent predictors of need for substance abuse treatment included use of cocaine/crack, living in the city of St. Louis at time of enrollment, and prescribed HAART in 1997. In this model, 85.2% of the cases were correctly classified. Women who were prescribed HAART in 1997 were less likely to have been identified as needing substance abuse treatment, and women who had a history of cocaine/crack use and who lived in the city of St. Louis were more likely to have been identified as needing substance abuse treatment.

In the model identifying predictors of prescribed HAART in 1997, we controlled for nadir CD4 counts and then allowed the remaining variables to enter in a stepwise fashion. A history of substance abuse was not related to prescription of HAART in 1997. African Americans compared to Caucasians

TABLE 3. Multiple Logistic Regression Analyses of Need for Substance Abuse Treatment and Prescription of HAART in 1997 and 1998

Variables[1]	Total R^2 at Entry[a]	O.R. (95% C.I.)	Significance of log LR
Need for Substance Abuse Treatment[b]			
Cocaine/crack abuse history	.362	19.65 (7.86-49.15)	.0000
Prescribed HAART in 1997	.417	0.18 (0.05-0.70)	.0055
In city of St. Louis at enrollment	.450	3.05 (1.18-7.85)	.0166
Prescribed HAART in 1997[c]			
Nadir CD4 count	.117	3.39 (1.76-6.50)	
Race	.237	0.23 (0.10-0.55)	.0008
Quarterly medical visits in 1997 (No.)	.308	1.80 (1.21-2.68)	.0015
Minutes/intervention (No.)	.343	0.95 (0.91-0.99)	.0181
Prescribed HAART in 1998[d]			
Prescribed HAART in 1997		22.15 (7.00-70.05)	
Nadir CD4 count	.408	1.40 (0.80-2.45)	
Quarterly medical visits in 1997	.458	1.66 (1.18-2.35)	.0019
Need for substance abuse treatment	.500	0.16 (0.04-0.62)	.0020

Notes
[1] In order of entry.
O.R. = odds ratio. 95% C.I. = 95% confidence interval. log LR = log likelihood-ratio statistic.
[a] Nagelkerke R^2
[b] N = 202 (subset of respondents with complete data).
[c] N = 199; two Hispanic respondents and one woman without CD4 data were excluded from analysis.
[d] N = 201; one woman without CD4 data was excluded from analysis.

and women who had less time per intervention with a case manager or social worker were less likely to be prescribed HAART in 1997. Adherence with quarterly medical visits was associated with prescribed HAART in 1997. This model correctly classified 81.4% of the cases.

In the model identifying predictors of use of HAART in 1998, we controlled for nadir CD4 counts and use of HAART in 1997. In this model, 80.6% of the cases were correctly classified. Adherence with quarterly medical visits was associated with prescription of HAART in 1998. Women identified as needing substance abuse treatment, however, were less likely to be prescribed HAART in 1998.

DISCUSSION

This study has several findings worth highlighting. First, a rigorous evaluation method identified a greater prevalence of substance abuse history among these Midwestern women than initially anticipated. Over 74% of the women were past or current substance abusers (excluding tobacco smoking). Over half had abused alcohol and marijuana, and nearly one-third had used cocaine. These rates of substance abuse history are higher than those reported for the 1996 United States general population over the age of 12, especially for use of cocaine (31.2% vs. 10.3%), marijuana (58.4% vs. 32%), heroin (9.4% vs. 1.1%), and amphetamines (7.5% vs. 2.3%). Interestingly, a history of tobacco smoking was lower in our group than in the general population (61.4% vs. 71.6%; Smith, Lundy, & Givel, 1998). However, like other studies (Bien & Burge, 1990; Burling & Ziff, 1988; Sussman, Dent, & Galaif, 1997), we found that tobacco smoking co-occurred with abuse of alcohol and other drugs. In addition, substance abuse behaviors were more likely to be found in the older women, similar to national figures (Smith et al., 1998). History of IDU was low among the women enrolled at HHSCC (12.3% total), with 22 (7.1%) reporting IDU as the mode of HIV infection. This low rate was anticipated as St. Louis metropolitan surveillance reports indicate that only 16% of the women currently living with HIV reported IDU as a primary risk factor for HIV infection (G. Harvey, personal communication, December 23, 1998).

Of concern, we found that only 43.9% of those women identified as needing substance abuse treatment had received such treatment. Potential reasons for this unmet need include: women may be unwilling to accept that they have a substance abuse problem, are not ready to undergo therapy, and have a paucity of substance abuse treatment programs and support available, especially for those with young children (Weissman, Melchior, Huba, Altice, Booth, Cottler, Genser, Jones, McCarthy, Needle, & Smereck, 1995). However, we found that a substance abuse history was positively correlated with the number of interventions and time spent with a nurse, nurse practitioner, case manager, and/or social worker. Thus having a history of abuse of various substances was, in fact, associated with a greater number of nurse/social work-case management interventions, even though the majority of these interventions were not directly related to substance abuse treatment. However, women needing substance abuse treatment were less likely to have been prescribed HAART in 1998.

With regard to medical care visits, the majority (72%) of women came to the comprehensive care clinic in 1997 less frequently than the recommended quarterly visits per the current guidelines (Carpenter, Fischl, Hammer et al., 1998; Report of the NIH Panel, 1998). In the linear regression model, adherence with quarterly medical visits in 1997 was associated with prescription of HAART, alcohol abuse history, and nursing interventions. In assessment by multiple logistic regressions, adherence with quarterly medical follow-up was associated with prescription of HAART in both 1997 and 1998, but not associated with the need for substance abuse treatment. The association of prescribing of HAART with medical clinic visits is not surprising, since close clinical monitoring is required for that complex treatment.

Since we were unable to distinguish between women who were currently abusing various substances and those who were not, we are unable to distinguish the relationships of these behaviors with utilization of various medical and social services. In a report about antiretroviral therapy among IDUs, Celentano, Vlahov, Cohn, Shadle, Obasanjo, and Moore (1998) reported that prior use is not the same as current substance use. In that study, abstinence from substance use and stable living conditions were associated with prescription of antiretroviral therapy, but not with the protease inhibitor based regimens. Of all the substances we evaluated, history of cocaine/crack use was positively associated with the need for substance abuse treatment, and, in turn, the need for substance abuse treatment was negatively associated with HAART prescription in 1998 (Table 3). Since at least one other study has identified a lack of association of substance abuse history with non-adherence to protease inhibitor therapy (Bangsberg, Tulsky, Hecht, & Moss, 1997), we are undergoing further evaluation of this finding.

Among study limitations, we recognize that the 74% prevalence rate of current or ever substance abuse is an overestimate of the actual need for substance abuse treatment in this population. We believe that the 18% of patients identified as needing substance abuse treatment is a more accurate reflection of current need. Second, we sampled only women receiving services at an HIV care facility in the St. Louis area, thus these data may not be able to be generalized to other sites. Third, our data on prescription of HAART were not linked with the biological responses to combination therapies; these analyses are underway. Finally, most of our data were based on patient self-reports.

The implications of this study are numerous. First, communities serving women with HIV need to be sensitive to the risks and impact of substance abuse, before and after HIV transmission. Second, there is ongoing debate as to the feasibility of engaging substance abusers in HAART, especially since failure to adhere to these complex regimens can limit future therapeutic options and increase resistant viral strains within the general community (Deeks, Smith, Holodniy, & Kahn, 1997; Bartlett, 1998). Some studies have shown higher rates of non-adherence among substance abusers (Barbour; 1998; Besch, Morse, Simon, Hodges, & Franchino, 1997; Flanigan et al., 1998, Hirschhorn et al., 1998; Rabkin & Chesney, 1998) while other reports show that substance abuse is not predictive of non-adherence (Belzer, Fuchs, Tucker, & Slonimsky, 1998; Besch et al., 1997; Gourevitch, 1996). Over time, our staff has recognized that substance abuse is a factor to be considered when discussing motivation to adhere to antiretroviral therapy, evaluating medical complications during hospital admissions, and during perinatal care. Third, the regional diversity of our patients (Figure 1) reveals an additional challenge for our staff to provide services that are tailored for women living in diverse urban, suburban, and rural areas. Fourth, comprehensive HIV care programs may want to consider assessment of substance abuse and treatment referrals as continuous quality improvement indicators in patient- and program-level evaluations. Finally, these data have led us to redesign our method of initial and annual assessments of substance abuse. At enrollment, the case manager now completes this evaluation and files a summary into the medical record for coordination of treatment with the medical team. This change in infrastructure has several advantages: (1) it is a simple, ongoing, and uniform method for collecting the data; (2) it identifies substance abuse behaviors over 12 month intervals; and (3) it assesses the degree of dependency associated with the specific substances, using definitions from the National Institute of Drug Abuse (1998), to enhance plans for treatment or referral. Still, this revised substance abuse assessment method has not yet been validated and, as before, relies predominantly on self-report.

In summary, substance abuse history was unexpectedly high among this Midwest cohort of women with HIV enrolled in our program. Substance abuse issues continue to pose challenges for healthcare providers in terms of assessment for medical complications and HIV medication decision-making. It is important that providers have a system in place to evaluate the presence and severity of drug-specific abuse. Such infrastructure should allow for adequate substance abuse treatment to be integrated into comprehensive HIV care.

ACKNOWLEDGMENTS

The authors express their gratitude to those who assisted in this evaluation, namely the women enrolled at HHSCC, the HHSCC clinical staff (Rebecca Bathon, Tameshia Bridges, Ariel Burgess, Debra DeMarco, Laura Ellison, Debbie Gase, and Bridgette Sims) and the HHSCC evaluation staff (Don Hardin and Cherie Hill). In addition, the authors wish to thank Tanya Brown, Ryan White Title I Mental Health Coordinator, for providing substance abuse statistics and program assistance, John Holste for technical assistance, and The Measurement Group for the compilation of Module 2B and Module 24 data.

REFERENCES

Barbour, C. (1998). *Improved survival in HIV/AIDS patients treated with aggressive combination antiretroviral therapy* [Abstract]. International Conference on AIDS, 12, 1106.

Bangsberg, D., Tulsky, J., Hecht, F., & Moss, A. (1997). Protease inhibitors in the homeless. *JAMA, 278,* 63-65.

Bardequez, A., Wesley, Y., Grandchamp, J., Gaines, G., & Newsome, H. (1995). *The prenatal HIV/AIDS clinic (PHC): Three years experience with a novel approach to care for HIV-infected pregnant women* [Abstract]. HIV Infected Women's Conference, S53.

Bartlett J. G. (1998). *HIV Combination Antiretroviral Therapy II: Cost Issues* [Panel Discussion]. 126th Annual Meeting of the American Public Health Association. Washington DC, Abstract 2198.

Belzer, M., Fuchs, D., Tucker, D., & Slonimsky, G. (1998). *High risk behaviors are not predictive of anti-retroviral non-adherence in HIV-positive youth* [Abstract]. International Conference on AIDS, 12, 596.

Besch, C. L., Morse, E., Simon, P., Hodges, J., & Franchino, B. (1997). *Preliminary results of a compliance study within CPCRA 007 combination nucleoside study (NuCombo)* [Abstract]. 4th Conference Retroviruses and Opportunistic Infections, 111.

Bien, T. H., & Burge, R. (1990). Smoking and drinking: A review of the literature. *International Journal of the Addictions, 25* (12), 1429-1454.

Burling, T. A., & Ziff, D. C. (1988). Tobacco smoking: A comparison between alcohol and drug abuse inpatients. *Addictive Behaviors, 13,* 185-190.

Carpenter, C. C., Fischl, M. A., Hammer, S. M. et al. (1998). Antiretroviral therapy for HIV infection in 1998: Updated recommendations of the International AIDS Society-USA Panel. *JAMA, 280,* 78-86.

Celetano, D. D., Vlahov, D., Cohn, S., Shadle, V. M., Obasanjo, O., & Moore, R. D. (1998). Self-reported antiretroviral therapy in injection drug users. *JAMA, 280* (6), 544-546.

Centers for Disease Control and Prevention. (1997). Update; trends in AIDS incidence–United States, 1996. *Morbidity and Mortality Weekly Report, 46* (37), 861-867.

Deeks, S. G., Smith, M., Holodniy, M., & Kahn, J. O. (1997). HIV-1 protease inhibitors. A review for clinicians. *JAMA, 277* (2), 145-153.

Flanigan, T. P., Merriman, N., Dickinson, B. P., Fiore, T., Tashima, K., Mitty, J., & Carpenter, C. C. (1998). *The effect of highly active antiretroviral therapy (HAART) and predictors of undetectable plasma viral loads in 250 HIV (+) women in care* [Abstract]. International Conference on AIDS, 12, 337.

Gourevitch, M. N. (1996). *Integrating primary care with substance abuse treatment: new standard?* [Abstract]. AHSR & FHSR Annual Meeting Abstract Book, 13, 148-149.

Hirschhorn, L., Quinones, J., Goldin, S., & Metras, L. (1998). *Highly active antiretroviral therapy (HAART) in the "real world": Experiences in an inner-city community health center (CHC).* [Abstract]. International Conference on AIDS, 12, 588.

Huba, G. J., Melchior, L. A., Staff of The Measurement Group, and the HRSA SPNS Program Cooperative Agreement Projects (1997a). *Module 2B: Intervention-Services Form.* Available: www.TheMeasurementGroup.com.

Huba, G. J., Melchior, L. A., Staff of The Measurement Group, and the HRSA SPNS Program Cooperative Agreement Projects (1997b). *Module 24: Brief Substance Abuse History Form.* Available: www.TheMeasurementGroup.com.

National Institute of Drug Abuse. *Criteria for substance dependence diagnosis.* (1998). www.nida.nih.gov. National Institute of Health.

Nelson, W. L., Ferrando, S. J, Stanislawski, D. M., & Garcia, P. M. (1996). *Childhood trauma, substance abuse, and distress in HIV-infected women* [Abstract]. International Conference on AIDS, 11, 429.

Rabkin, J. G., & Chesney, M. A. (1998). Adhering to complex regimens for HIV. *GMHC Treatment Issues, 12*(4), 1-9.

Report of the NIH Panel to Define Principles of Therapy of HIV Infection. (1998). *Annals of Internal Medicine, 128*, 1057-1078.

Smith, R. C., Lundy, C. J., & Givel, M. S. (1998). *Status report on Missouri's alcohol and drug abuse problems.* Jefferson City, MO: Missouri Department of Mental Health, Division of Alcohol and Drug Abuse, Jefferson City, MO.

SPSS 8.0.2 [Computer Software]. (1997). Chicago. IL: SPSS Inc.

Sussman, S., Dent, C. W., & Galaif, E. R. (1997). The correlates of substance abuse and dependence among adolescents at high risk for drug abuse. *Journal of Substance Abuse, 9*, 241-255.

Weissman, G., Melchior, L., Huba, G., Altice, R., Booth, R., Cottler, L., Genser, S., Jones, S., McCarthy, S., Needle, R., & Smereck, G. (1995). Women living with substance abuse and HIV disease: Medical care access issues. *Journal of the American Medical Women's Association, 50*, 115-120.

Issues in Implementing and Evaluating a Managed Care Home Health Care System for HIV/AIDS: Visiting Nurse Association Foundation of Los Angeles

David A. Cherin, PhD
G. J. Huba, PhD
Lisa A. Melchior, PhD
Susan Enguidanos, MPH
W. June Simmons, LCSW
Diana E. Brief, PhD

SUMMARY. Blending curative and palliative orientations to care in the home care services delivery of terminal HIV/AIDS patients pro-

David A. Cherin was affiliated with the Visiting Nurse Association Foundation, Los Angeles, CA at the time this was written. He is now affiliated with the University of Washington School of Social Work, Seattle, WA. G. J. Huba, and Lisa A. Melchior are associated with The Measurement Group, Culver City, CA. Susan Enguidanos and W. June Simmons are affiliated with the Visiting Nurse Association Foundation, Los Angeles, CA. The late Diana E. Brief was affiliated with The Measurement Group, Culver City, CA.

Address correspondence to: David A. Cherin, PhD, University of Washington School of Social Work, 4101 15th Avenue NE, Office 127b, Seattle, WA 98121.

This work was supported in part by the Health Resources and Services Administration (HRSA), HIV/AIDS Bureau (HAB), Special Projects of National Significance (SPNS) Grant No. 5 U90 HA 00044-05. This publication's contents are solely the responsibility of the authors and do not necessarily represent the official view of the funding agency.

[Haworth co-indexing entry note]: "Issues in Implementing and Evaluating a Managed Care Home Health System for HIV/AIDS: Visiting Nurse Association Foundation of Los Angeles." Cherin, David A. et al. Co-published simultaneously in *Drugs & Society* (The Haworth Press, Inc.) Vol. 16, No. 1/2, 2000, pp. 203-222; and: *Evaluating HIV/AIDS Treatment Programs: Innovative Methods and Findings* (ed: G. J. Huba et al.) The Haworth Press, Inc., 2000, pp. 203-222. Single or multiple copies of this article are available for a fee from The Haworth Document Delivery Service [1-800-342-9678, 9:00 a.m. - 5:00 p.m. (EST). E-mail address: getinfo@haworthpressinc.com].

duces a cost efficient and patient effective overall model of care. This article characterizes the development, implementation, and evaluation of the Visiting Nurse Association Foundation of Los Angeles' (VNAF-LA) Transprofessional Model of terminal home care. Palliatively trained social workers were made part of the VNAF-LA's regular home care service delivery teams to create a biopsychosocial perspective to pre-hospice terminal care services. This enrollment to routine home care produced significant cost reductions and improved patients' quality of life. In addition, evaluation data were used to develop a cost profile of patient care. *[Article copies available for a fee from The Haworth Document Delivery Service: 1-800-342-9678. E-mail address: <getinfo@haworth pressinc.com> Website: <http://www.HaworthPress.com>]*

KEYWORDS. Home care, terminal care, HIV/AIDS, managed care, palliative care, evaluation

INTRODUCTION

The *Capitated Care for End-stage HIV/AIDS Patients* Project of the Visiting Nurse Association Foundation of Los Angeles (VNAF-LA) aims to develop and evaluate a capitated model of home and hospice care for end-stage AIDS patients. This is a salient issue given the increase in survival time of people with HIV/AIDS resulting from new medications and combination therapies. To meet the increasing need for capitated care for people with HIV/AIDS, the VNAF-LA project designed a capitation model (sub-contract to primary health care providers for home care services) of reimbursement that is specifically applicable to AIDS home care issues and the removal of barriers that facilitate continuity of care through more timely and appropriate utilization of hospice palliative treatment care and case management.

The VNAF-LA's continuity of care model has resulted in numerous program achievements in providing home care and hospice services to HIV/AIDS patients. The model developed preliminary capitation rates and produced nearly ten percent lower costs than traditional home care models and found that clients in the continuity of care model experienced a higher quality of life than clients in traditional home care. The project also demonstrated that a psychosocial orientation in home care is more efficient and more effective than a pure medical orientation in home care. This validated the continuity of care model to be more cost efficient and more effective in meeting patient needs.

The innovative model bridges the gap between palliative and curative services through utilization of hospice-trained nurses and social workers as case managers and care providers in the entire episode of a patient's home care. This hospice team introduces into the home care, the medical-surgical care arena, cost management techniques, training in a biopsychosocial model of patient care, and a focus on the patient. An integrated model of service delivery, which is based on interdisciplinary, care management and blended modalities of service, provides a cost-effective method in the provision of home care services for terminally ill AIDS patients (Cherin, Huba, Brief & Melchior, 1998), especially given the range of psychosocial issues–such as substance abuse–present for many persons with HIV/AIDS (Melchior, De-Veauuse, & Huba, 1998).

This study presents significant policy implications for the future of end-stage care and services for HIV/AIDS patients specifically, and perhaps terminal chronic care in general. The study proved that introducing a blended model of care into the mainstream of terminal care has significant effects in reducing costs and for the development of a capitated community-based model of treatment. By slightly altering the care team to be inclusive of biopsychosocial issues, the profile of service delivery and the costs of service delivery are substantially changed.

The research literature is scant in reporting evaluation studies of HIV home care and hospice services. Some home care counseling programs have been evaluated using qualitative methods (e.g., Buwalda, Kruijthoff, de Bruyn, & Hogewoning, 1994; Melchior, DeVeauuse, & Huba, 1998). Care-giver characteristics have been studied to examine the effects of satisfaction and stress on behaviors of home health care workers on AIDS patients (Ferrari, McCown, & Pantano, 1993). However, the effects of enhanced models of end stage AIDS care have not been extensively evaluated. Thus the present study represents a unique contribution to this important literature.

Medicaid and legislative environment. Due to rising health costs, traditional fee-for-service in the United States is being replaced by financial reimbursement based on utilization review and capitated payments. Federal and State programs such as Medicare and Medicaid are turning toward managed care in an attempt to control rising costs (Gamliel, Politzer, Rivo & Mullan, 1995). Almost all states are in the process of moving Medicaid enrollees, including those with HIV, into managed care (Gamliel, Singer & Marconi, 1998). California is actively seeking to enroll MediCal patients in Health Maintenance Organizations and is a 1915b waiver state, which allows waiving provisions regarding freedom of provider choice to beneficiaries. There are currently no home care companies, private or public, that are managed care primary providers. All home care organizations actively subcontract with primary care providers to provide the broad array of home care services to HIV/AIDS patients inclusive of intravenous therapy, medical-surgical services, and hospice services.

HIV Issues in Managed Care

Home care services for HIV/AIDS patients have until recently been primarily focused on intravenous services and medical-surgical services directed towards medication management. As a consequence of this limited experience, many of the home care agencies in California have a limited database available to calculate and understand the capitation of the full spectrum of home care services. HIV/AIDS patients, beyond medical-surgical care, with the advent of protease inhibitor therapy, often require psychosocial services (social work) as well as sustained medical nursing care. In addition, few home care agencies understand the need for blending of curative and palliative services required for HIV/AIDS patients. Home care companies are at a distinct disadvantage in costs, contracting and providing home care services.

Most HIV/AIDS patient care is delivered by managed care companies on a Medicare model, a discounted fee for service reimbursement system. Services are case managed with a view by the case manager of justifying and certifying single service encounters. The difficulty with this model of service delivery is that care provided to HIV/AIDS patients is not episodic, incident by incident, but rather runs a long trajectory over the course of the illness. Therefore, health care for patients with HIV/AIDS needs to be managed over time, as opposed to being viewed as a single episode of care. The care management model, in opposition to a fee for service model of care as validated by the VNAF-LA capitated home care model, is designed for the managed care environment. Care management requires a view of the entire combined episodes of care and is based on cross training of home care services delivery personnel.

Improvements in medical treatment inclusive of new pharmacological regimens (combination therapies, protease inhibitors) have enabled many AIDS patients to live longer and many to return from certified hospice programs. The impact of these changes has altered the course of AIDS care significantly. Protease inhibitors also have raised a host of issues about reforming the continuum of care and service delivery for AIDS patients. One of the more profound changes in the continuum of care for AIDS patients centers on end-stage care, hospice, and its utilization. Certified hospice programs, like the VNAF-LA/Sun Alliance in-home hospice programs, are the only care venues at this time that provide an active and continuous combination of palliative and curative services. However, patients must be certified as having six months or less to live before they can be admitted to hospice programs.

Models of care. The VNAF-LA project compares two service models for providing home healthcare services to individuals in the late stages of AIDS care. The two models are a capitated model of care, the Transprofessional Model, which is a blended care model, and the Standard Model of traditional home care nursing. Figure 1 compares the major characteristics of the two models utilized by the VNAF-LA project. In the Transprofessional Model, services are coordinated, primarily through the use of a case manager, to develop an integrated system of blended care. In the Standard Model, the patient may receive services from the same medical and social work professionals, but the individual providers are not closely blended into a treatment team. Thus, as compared to the Standard Model, the Transprofessional Model is one in which a team approach to treatment is the centerpiece, giving various professionals a more complete view of the individual patient.

Current literature and research on terminal care, specifically on AIDS, indicates that the nature of AIDS terminal care requires a mixing of treatment orientations, including palliative and curative services, to help patients meet biological, psychological, and social needs by assisting them to participate in

FIGURE1. Comparison of Two Models*

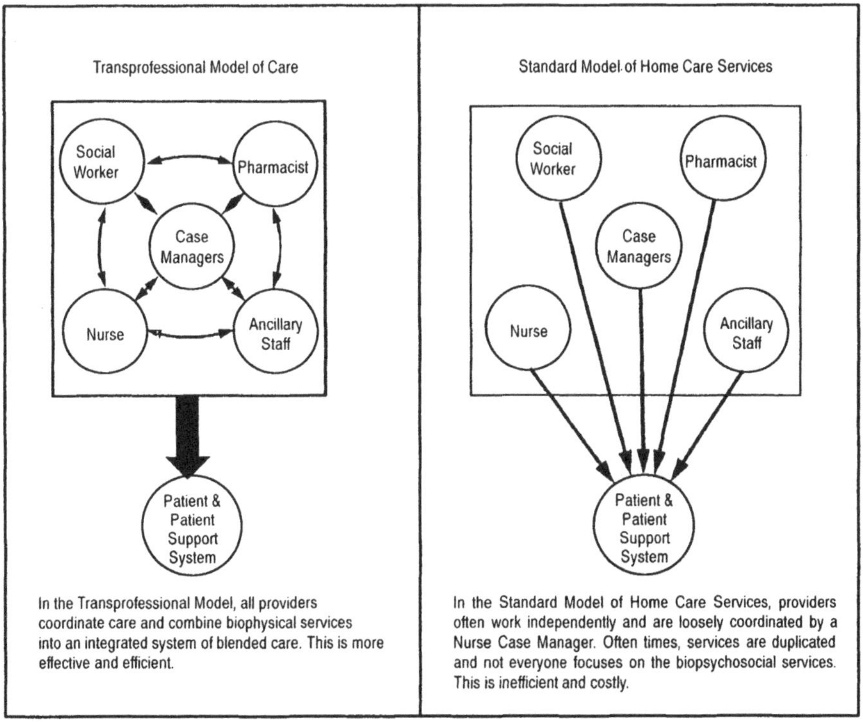

Transprofessional Model of Care

In the Transprofessional Model, all providers coordinate care and combine biophysical services into an integrated system of blended care. This is more effective and efficient.

Standard Model of Home Care Services

In the Standard Model of Home Care Services, providers often work independently and are loosely coordinated by a Nurse Case Manager. Often times, services are duplicated and not everyone focuses on the biopsychosocial services. This is inefficient and costly.

*Figure taken from Cherin, D. A., Huba, G. J., Brief, D. E., & Melchior, L. A. (1998). Evaluation of the transprofessional model of home health care for HIV/AIDS. *Home Health Care Services Quarterly, 17* (1), 55-72.

their own care and treatment decisions. The service utilization profile of terminally ill AIDS patients can be used to evaluate more precisely the service areas in which cost for patient services differ. Individuals assigned to the experimental Transprofessional Model demonstrated a different service utilization profile than those assigned to a Traditional Model of care. Patients assigned to the Transprofessional Model tended to receive the average number of visits per day for most service categories, while those in the Traditional Model received more home health aide and IV nurse visits (Cherin, Huba, Brief, & Melchior, 1998). Rather than hospice being an ancillary modality in the arsenal of the medical model of care, palliation and psychosocial care need to be integrated into end-stage treatment throughout the treatment process (Anderson & MacElveen-Hoehn, 1988; Foley, Flannery, Grayton, Flintoft, & Cook, 1995). This implies that the route to potential cost savings in AIDS terminal care is through a fully integrated model of care that is not dichotomized between curative and palliative services.

In response to the paradox in terminal care presented by AIDS, the VNAF-LA project's research effort is designed to evaluate the effectiveness of the blending of palliative and curative treatments throughout terminal care using a managed care framework at its base. Rather than continue to explore the efficiency of palliative care over acute care in the terminal phase of patient treatment, the current model was designed to introduce a managed, blended model of care, featuring both a curative and palliative treatment focus throughout the period of care for terminal patients, and to develop a capitated service delivery and reimbursement model of care in a community-based home care setting.

The target population for this research was late-stage AIDS patients who reside in the catchment area of the Visiting Nurse Association of Los Angeles (VNAF-LA/Regency). This area encompasses most of Los Angeles County, including the San Fernando Valley, South Central Los Angeles, Hollywood, and the coastal cities; the Antelope Valley, the San Gabriel Valley; and patients who have been referred to the VNAF-LA/Regency from Los Angeles County-USC Medical Center, AIDS Healthcare Foundation (AHF), Health Care Partners, Kaiser Permanente, and private physician offices and clinics. Based on the patients served in the first three years of this study, the demographic profile of the population in service with the VNAF-LA Transprofessional Model was predominantly Caucasian (44.5 percent), and male (86.0 percent), with a mean age of 38.1 years ($SD = 10.1$ years). Approximately 33.5 percent of the sample was Latino and 18.0 percent was African American.

Fiscal issues and benefits (services). In general usage, the concept of capitation applies to a somewhat different healthcare delivery approach than that followed by the VNAF-LA. Specifically, a capitation reimbursement approach causes one or more of the participants in the healthcare delivery system, such as the managed care organization (MCO), individual or group practice provider, or ancillary service provider, to bear risk for the level of utilization and for the unit cost of services provided to a select population. In return for accepting the risk, the MCO (which is used here as short hand for all risk bearing entities) has the right to perform pre-authorization of services, utilization management, case management, provider profiling, and selection. It develops network discounting arrangements and uses other managed care tools. The client population group is defined simply to be that group of individuals who are eligible for services from the MCO.

In order to bear the risk inherent in capitation reimbursement, the MCO must determine the likely level of healthcare utilization and unit costs and how those levels can be controlled using the management tools available. However, those estimates are inherently uncertain, especially if the capitation reimbursement approach and the managed care techniques are being instituted for the first time. Further, the uncertainty cannot be determined from actuarial averages and standards, but can be determined using statistical estimation. For example, an MCO may project inpatient admissions at 75 per thousand lives and the average length of stay at 5 days per admission under its planned utilization management approach. However, in looking at its previous contracts, it determines that the admissions actually range from 65 to 80 per thousand and the average length of stay ranges from 4.2 to 6.0 days for a similar population (after adjusting its other population groups to be compatible with the age and sex characteristics of the group under consideration). In this case, the company can estimate statistically the likelihood that the utilization will exceed 75 admissions per thousand and an average length of stay of 5 days, which is the uncertainty that the company must offset.

Typically, MCOs deal with this uncertainty in several ways. First, stop-loss insurance can be obtained to limit the MCO's loss to certain dollar amounts over the projected baseline cost. Second, the MCO can create a reserve (usually around 2.0 percent) in its pricing to cover part of the potential losses. Third, the MCO can simply adjust its utilization and unit cost projections slightly upward to cover part of the loss, such as using 77 or 78 admissions per thousand instead of 75. Fourth, the MCO may create a tiered capitation approach, in which the occurrence of a specified utilization will result in an add-on to the base price, thereby relieving the MCO of some or all of the risk. Fifth, the MCO may simply not take risk for certain circumstances–such as particular diagnoses–but simply treat them on a fee-for-service basis.

In order to be competitive, various combinations of these strategies can be examined and traded off in order to minimize price for a given level of risk, or minimize risk at a certain competitive price. For example, over certain ranges of projected utilization and cost, stop-loss insurance premiums may be relatively constant, then drop dramatically if the MCO bears slightly more risk internally. Identifying these pricing break points and comparing the pricing impact to other risk offsets can lead to a more competitive price.

Capitation by the VNAF-LA: A case rate approach. The VNAF-LA capitation model differs from most commercial capitation models in several important ways. In contrast to commonly used commercial managed care organization (MCO) approaches, the VNAF-LA capitation approach establishes eligibility on the basis of a disease diagnosis (HIV-positive or full-blown AIDS) and accepts the risk for the home healthcare treatment of those diseases. That is, the VNAF-LA does not accept the risk of a certain number of random individuals in a client base contracting HIV/AIDS, as would a commercial MCO, but enrolls only those individuals who already have contracted the disease.

The VNAF-LA capitation approach also differs from a carve out type of capitation in which the MCO accepts the risk of an individual contracting a disease within a general population group, but only for a particular disease such as cancer. Although the carve out approach does deal with a single disease, it is still based on the risk of a covered eligible person contracting the disease and needing to be treated. This is in contrast to the VNAF-LA capitation approach of accepting only the risk of treatment, not the risk of contracting a specific disease in a general population group.

One can think of the different capitation approaches in a vertical hierarchy of risk. At the bottom level of a pyramid, an MCO would accept the risk of an eligible person contracting any diseases and providing disease treatment for all covered eligibles. At the next level up, the MCO accepts the risk of eligibles contracting and of the MCO treating a specific disease for all covered lives, i.e., a carve out type of coverage. This is a narrower and more specialized capitation coverage. At the highest (and narrowest) level in the pyramid, the MCO does not accept the risk of eligibles contracting a disease, but only of disease treatment, and then only for a particular disease. This case rate approach is the narrowest and most specialized capitation coverage and corresponds to the VNAF-LA capitation approach.

The fact that VNAF-LA is at the top of the risk hierarchy means that it does not have to consider the factors associated with eligibles contracting a disease (HIV/AIDS), but only those factors associated with disease treatment. Instead of an exposure matrix to project the likely number of cases contracted per 100,000 individuals, the VNAF-LA capitation approach focuses on treatment parameters such as days on service and types of treatment (an intensity of services model). In essence, the VNAF-LA capitation approach is a case rate, disease care management approach, with the VNAF-LA accepting risk for the length and intensity of treatment provided to eligibles.

The concept of a risk pyramid is used to compare and distinguish the VNAF-LA capitation approach from the commercial concepts of full capitation and carve out capitation. It also indicates how the approach the VNAF-LA must take to capitation development and risk bearing differs from the other two approaches. First, the VNAF-LA capitation approach involves less risk in the sense that the VNAF-LA does not have to develop an exposure matrix and then project the contracted number of cases of one or more diseases in its population group based on the actuarial data for a group with the particular age, sex, income and other characteristics. The VNAF-LA does not need, for example, to develop underwriting factors based on a population group. Second, the VNAF-LA needs to address only the risk associated with a specific disease (HIV/AIDS), as opposed to dealing with numerous diseases and the associated differences in provider recruitment and utilization management. Third, the population group covered by the VNAF-LA HRSA SPNS Program demonstration project consists of those individuals on home healthcare and those individuals in home hospice, both of whom have reasonably well defined treatment profiles, days on service, intensity of service, and survival curves. Therefore, from a statistical viewpoint, the VNAF-LA population group has less statistical diversity and uncertainty than would a full capitation or carve out eligible population.

Although the VNAF-LA population group presents less risk to capitation than does a general population group, as described above, it also presents several potential sources of greater risk. First, all of the VNAF-LA client population has contracted HIV and suffers a variety of symptoms associated with the different disease clusters. Therefore, there is no base of healthy clients who do not need treatment, such as in a full capitation population group. Second, and of central importance to this analysis, treatment regimens are presently changing in such a way as to dramatically lengthen the period of survival (and treatment) for a large segment of the VNAF-LA population group.

If multi-drug therapies involving protease inhibitors can be expected to be effective for sixty percent of the population and if these treatments extend the survival rates dramatically–both reasonable assumptions at this point–the uncertainty in projected days on service could increase sharply and the intensity of treatment could also decrease. Unfortunately, at this point there is no evidence sufficient to estimate the extent of these two effects.

Within the VNAF-LA's healthcare delivery model–treatment of HIV/ AIDS in a home healthcare program–capitation in fact means case rate capitation, as opposed to the full capitation or carve out capitation that is seen in most managed care organizations. Although this approach involves less risk than the more general approaches, it still entails considerable risk.

Case rate capitation methodology. The research methodology utilized in studying the VNAF-LA approach is based upon the case rate capitation concept described above. As stated previously, under the case rate capitation approach, the VNAF-LA is not at risk for the rate of contraction of HIV or of the conversion of HIV-positive persons to full blown AIDS for a client population group; it is at risk for the treatment of the disease once the client has entered the program. Therefore, no actuarial analysis of random population groups is required, nor is there a need to develop underwriting factors for such a population group. (However, as described above, it is likely that underwriting will be required based upon the use of drug therapies that use protease inhibitors in combination with other drugs.)

Under case rate capitation, the VNAF-LA home care services and other home care companies contracting in a managed care environment are at risk for three factors: (1) Duration of home care (the length of time a patient remains in the home healthcare program); (2) Intensity (the intensity/mix of the home care services); and (3) Cost (the unit and the total cost of the treatment).

The first risk variable, duration of home care, is clear conceptually, but it raises certain measurement problems. First, some patients may enter the program, leave, and enter again, displaying an episodic participation and utilization pattern. One could measure their length of time in the program as either the sum of all the periods in which they actively received services, or as the time from their initial entry into the program until their final exit, such as into hospice or through death. Under a case rate capitation approach, it is envisioned that the capitation rate is applied much as a lifetime benefit in an insurance policy, providing a total benefit amount. As a result, the time from initial entry to final exit from the program would be the actual risk to the VNAF-LA, even if the patient left and re-entered the program several times. Therefore, the duration from initial entry to final exit is the appropriate measure of risk exposure for the VNAF-LA.

A second problem with the duration of home care variable is patients may exit the program for different reasons, not solely for entry into the hospice program. It is important to know the relative probabilities for each reason for exiting the home health program, whether it is to enter into hospice, due to death, or some other reason.

The third problem in accepting risk for the duration of home care is that combination drug therapies using protease inhibitors are leading to dramatic changes in the length of, and indeed the need for, home healthcare. This implies that under a case rate capitation, the VNAF-LA could now have responsibility for a much longer duration of treatment, although at a level of intensity that is likely to be somewhat lower. In fact, there is no sufficient evidence yet to suggest how much longer home care lasts when clients receive combination drug therapies. If the drug therapies continue to be successful, the treatment could evolve into a chronic care scenario as opposed to the time limited home healthcare program leading to hospice care. Given that there is not sufficient data to understand the full implications of combination drug therapies on the duration of home care, it is not possible for the VNAF-LA, or other home care agencies, to accept risk for the duration of treatment.

It is proposed to treat these combination drug therapies as an underwriting variable and to seek, when contracting, non-capitated reimbursement. That is, to the extent that a client finds the combination drug treatments to be effective, which may extend their duration of home care, the client no longer would be kept in the case rate capitation pool, but would be moved instead into a monthly capitation, based on a fixed monthly cost of treatment. This could also mean that the individual might have benefits remaining under the unused case rate capitation, which could be accessed at a later date.

Evaluation results from two models of home care services. The discussion of methodology for capitation development above defines the concept and rationale for the case rate capitation approach. This is a stronger approach than simply developing a monthly charge rate as other organizations have done; it also implies bearing risk over the full duration of delivery of home care services. The key risk factors are the duration of treatment, the intensity of treatment, and the unit cost of treatment.

Based on the key considerations discussed for development of a capitation case rate model, the following analysis is offered with regard to cost, units, and intensity of services. This analysis is offered as an example of case rate development.

For our most recent analyses of the data from the Transprofessional and Standard Model comparisons, we used the service records accumulated at the VNAF-LA through June 1997. Those service records represent 664 individuals and almost 6,601 days of services that project staff have added into the VNAF-LA central computerized management information system, which is also used to bill federal and local reimbursement agencies. After cleaning the data in a very extensive way and eliminating patients who were seen only one day (for enrollment services but who never followed through with full treatment regimens), we have a final, cleaned, fully-enrolled sample of 549 individuals available for analysis. Of these, 201 individuals received the Transprofessional Model and 348 received services under the Standard Model. The larger number of individuals in the Standard Model is due to the fact that the team responsible for the Transprofessional Model had a "full" case load in the later months of the study and the percentage of cases randomly assigned to them had to be lowered for this reason. [Note that our analyses of shift in randomization procedures indicate that this was not a confounding factor in any analyses; see Cherin, Huba, Brief, & Melchior, 1998.]

Our analyses indicate that the patients assigned to the Transprofessional and Standard Models are equivalent to one another on major demographic characteristics. For example, patients in the two conditions were not significantly different in terms of their gender, ages, ethnic backgrounds, primary language, or their primary medical insurance payer source. The average age of all patients was 38.67 years (*SD* = 9.10 years). The ethnic-racial composition of the patient base was 44.4 percent Caucasian, 20.0 percent African American, 34.1 percent Hispanic, and 1.5 percent Asian-Pacific Islander.

There were significant differences between the service arrays received by individuals under the two models and the costs of these services. Table 1 shows the average visit by service type per patient per day, received by individuals in each of the Transprofessional and Standard Models. In end-stage AIDS care, the most important cost element is that of IV nurse visits.

The 201 patients in the Transprofessional Model were seen by the VNAF-LA an average of 77.30 days (*SD* = 91.17 days), while the 348 patients in the Standard Model were seen an average of 78.07 days (*SD* = 107.78 days). The difference in days was statistically non-significant ($t = -.09, p > .9$).

Table 1 also looks at the types of services received, on the average, by members of the Transprofessional and Standard Model patient cohorts (we have converted scores to the metric of services per patient per day). Since most patients will not receive a service of a particular kind every day, numbers in this metric usually run in the range from 0 (indicating no services) to 1 (indicating the receipt of the service every day the patient was in treatment). Note that it is possible to receive more than one of each type of service per day, and for some types of services, such as IV Nursing, this may be the typical pattern rather than the exception. An empirical typology of these service patterns also differentiated the Transprofessional and Standard Models (Huba, Brief, Cherin, Panter, & Melchior, 1998).

In the column labeled "*t*-ratio for difference between visits per day" there are two numbers. The first number presented represents a *t*-test based on untransformed scores. In general, the distributions of these scores are decidedly non-normal. In order to make the scores more approximate the assumptions of parametric statistical testing, we transformed them using square root and logarithmic transformations to achieve distributions closer to the normal distribution. We looked at both sets of transformations and decided that the square root yielded a better approximation to a normal distribution curve. The second *t*-ratio in each cell is that for the transformation of the scores by the square root (first adding one to move all ratios to be greater or equal to one). In most cases the *t*-ratios calculated on raw or transformed scores are fairly identical and generally comparable. In one case (IV Nurse services) the *p* values for the statistical test jumped from .06 to .04, but it is an arbitrary distinction that one result is significant while one is not.

There is a significant difference in the average daily costs between the two

TABLE 1. Comparison of Two Models[1]

Visits by Service Type	Transprofessional Model		Standard Model		t-ratio for difference between visits per day	Ratio of daily costs in TP Model to S Model	Cost per patient per day under TP Model	Cost per patient per day under S Model	Difference in costs per patient per day(TP-S)
	Mean visits per patient per day	Standard deviation	Mean visits per patient per day	Standard deviation					
Public Health Nurse	.011	.046	.014	.115	−.44/−.29	.780	$.39	$.50	($.11)
Registered Nurse	.164	.337	.170	.329	−.21/−.22	.963	$5.65	$5.87	($.22)
LVN	.015	.123	.016	.078	−.08/−.25	.946	$.35	$.37	($.02)
Home Health Aide	.128	.412	.160	.400	−.90/−1.10	.797	$2.04	$2.56	($.52)
Physical Therapist	.019	.061	.022	.086	−.52/−.46	.848	$.89	$1.05	($.16)
Speech Therapist	.000	.006	.003	.030	−1.41/−1.42	.154	$.02	$.13	($.11)
Occupational Therapist	.001	.010	.008	.050	−2.23*/2.21*	.194	$.07	$.36	($.29)
MSW	.040	.088	.030	.090	1.23/1.39	1.316	$2.00	$1.52	$.48
IV Nurse	.092	.261	.141	.324	−1.93/−2.09	.656	$4.84	$7.38	($2.54)
Routine Healthcare	.008	.073	.002	.019	1.23/1.27	4.667	$.28	$.06	$.22
Holiday/After Hour	.000	.001	.001	.013	−.85/−.84	0.333	$.01	$.03	($.02)
Psychiatric Nurse	.006	.029	.010	.042	−1.50/−1.56	.549	$.28	$.51	($.23)
Evaluation Visit	.021	.086	.015	.048	.95/.93	1.417	$1.02	$.72	$.30
Extra Duty Nursing	.001	.005	.001	.010	−.90/−.89	.500	$.03	$.06	($.03)
Cardiac Nurse	.000	.001	.001	.024	−.94/−.93	.167	$.01	$.06	($.05)
Homemaker	.007	.048	.007	.060	−.15/−.19	.857	$.12	$.14	($.02)

*p < .05 **p < .01 ***p < .001

Note. The first t-test results are based on raw scores while the second t-test results are based on the square root transformation of the service units in order to stabilize the variances in the two groups. All t-test results given in this table and throughout this document do not assume that the variances in the two groups are the same (this is generally a more conservative test). The corresponding multivariate test of the entire array of services is significant (Wilks Λ = .868, p < .001). Costs associated with each service are based on standard cost multipliers established by the VNAF.

[1] Table taken from Cherin, D. A., Huba, G. J., Brief, D. E., & Melchior, L. A. (1998). Evaluation of the transprofessional model of home health care for HIV/AIDS. Home Health Care Services Quarterly, 17 (1), 55-72.

models of care. We have estimated that there is an average per patient per day cost of $17.99 under the Transprofessional Model and an average per patient per day cost of $21.30 under the Standard Model. The difference between the costs per patient per day are statistically significant ($t = -1.59$, $p < .06$ one-tailed for the untransformed data; $t = -2.44$, $p < .01$, one-tailed for data which have been transformed taking square roots). [One-tailed significance tests in this context are warranted as we clearly hypothesized in the original grant proposal that the Transprofessional Model would produce lower costs.] These daily rates translate to an average cost per patient of $1,543.95 under the Transprofessional Model and $1,675.46 under the Standard Model over an average treatment episode in each group. This represents a saving of $3.31 per patient per day or $131.51 per patient when the Transprofessional Model is used. Another way to state this is that there is a 7.85 percent saving in costs by moving the client to a Transprofessional Model.

Estimates of savings under the Transprofessional Model include staff time only and do not include pharmacy costs. In analysis of the data from the first year of pharmacy costs, it was found that the average pharmacy cost for patients receiving the Transprofessional Model was $2,258 while the cost for the patients under the Standard Model was $3,598, for an average cost savings of $1,340 under the Transprofessional Model.

There is another important outcome variable in the present analyses. We also calculated the Hospice Nurse visits for the patients in the Transprofessional Model and those in the Standard Model. Transprofessional patients had an average of .067 Hospice Nurse Visits per day ($SD = .155$) while Standard patients had an average of .005 visits ($SD = .027$). Transforming the scores using a square root transformation resulted in a significant difference between the conditions ($t = 5.70$, $p < .001$ without transformation; $t = 7.70$, $p < .001$, with the square root transformation). The Hospice Nurse visits when either the patient has indicated that it is time to be admitted to the hospice or when the clinical team feels that the patient should consider entering hospice care. We found that it is 14.56 times more likely that a Transprofessional Model patient will see a Hospice Nurse during the course of treatment than it is for a Standard Model patient. This outcome is viewed as direct evidence that the Transprofessional Model is having the desired result of moving patients into hospice as they accept the end-stage of the disease.

A second way to examine group differences is to use the analytic framework of a survival curve. This is a negative exponential function that describes how many individuals are still on service after each additional period of time. It can be thought of as the probability that an individual is still on service after a specified number of days. For example, the initial probability is 100 percent at day one. After 10 days, the probability may go down to, say, 95 percent. After several months it may decline to 50 percent. Similarly, one may think of the curve as it applies to a group of individuals. Of an initial cohort, the survival curve indicates what percentage of the group is still on service after a specified period of time. In other words, the curve describes a reduction profile for the initial group over time, as opposed to the probabilistic behavior of a single individual. The curve will be used in both ways in this analysis. (It should be noted parenthetically that survival curves are widely used in many applications from actuarial analysis and loss distributions to radioactive decay and half-life estimation in atomic particles.)

The importance of survival analysis is that it not only demonstrates the overall difference in average behavior, but it presents a more detailed picture. Figure 2 shows the traditional Kaplan-Meier survival curves for the members of the Transprofessional and Standard Model groups. These curves should be read as follows. The vertical (Y) axis shows the probability that a client will still be on service. The horizontal (X) axis shows the number of days in service. As can be seen, the two groups tend to have about the same curves for the first 10 months (300 days) but that the curves differ after that with the Transprofessional Model clients tending to leave the service (as they transition into hospice). Using traditional tests for the equality of survival curves, there is no statistical difference.

Just comparing the average length of time on service, as estimated from the survival analysis, we find that the average length is 112.2 days (standard error of 9.65 days) for the Transprofessional Model clients and 109.9 days (standard error of 8.36 days) for the Standard Model clients. The difference is not statistically significant. Note that the method of survival analysis uses information about censoring (or which clients remain on service at the time that data collection stops) in their estimates and that these numbers are somewhat different than those reported earlier that do not account for censoring. Note that the earlier estimates were also for total days of service as opposed to total time on service (or at risk for services).

If we examine the curves in Figure 2, it appears that the differences between the models appear after about 10 months when the Transprofessional Model clients are less likely to still remain on service. To test whether this was true, we fit a more sophisticated survival analysis using Cox regression. The "time dependent covariate" model fit specifically asks whether the curves are closer, or further apart, at different times. The model fit included the effects of experimental group, the gender of the client, the interaction of experimental group by gender, the interaction of experimental group by time, the interaction of gender by time, and the three-way interaction of experimental group by gender by time. Using a sequence of model entry in which the three-way interactions were added to the model, then the two-way interactions, and then the main effects, the only effects that were significant were that of the interaction of group by time (Wald statistic = 6.65, *d.f.* = 1, *p* <

FIGURE 2. Kaplan-Meier Survival Curves for the Members of the Transprofessional and Standard Model*

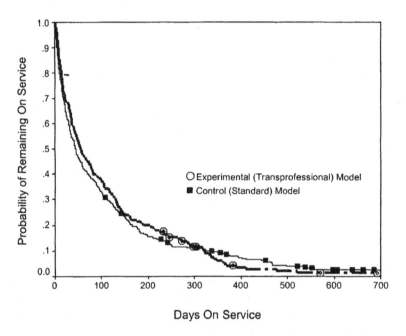

Days On Service

*Figure adapted from Huba, G. J., Cherin, D. A., & Melchior, L. A. (1998). Retention of clients in service under two models of home healthcare for HIV/AIDS. *Home Health Care Services Quarterly, 17* (3), 17-26.

.01). The two conditions differ in retention rates on service primarily for longer time periods. The gender by treatment group interaction was also significant (Wald statistic = 7.00, *d.f.* = 1, *p* < .01) with the difference being that women in the control group were the most likely to stay in the service for very long periods of time.

This finding is important from two points of view. First, the overall averages of the two groups do not reveal this difference. Second, the data suggest that the experimental program is most effective at the end of the home care period. The implications are clear: intervention through the Transprofessional care model is effective especially as the client nears death and should be transitioned into hospice.

The results indicate, using a case rate model, that the Transprofessional care approach would result in 27.0 percent savings per case. Applied to a total of 1,000 plus cases that the VNAF-LA SPNS project has served, the total cost reduction would be several million dollars, due to the use of the blended care model.

Cost control under the VNAF-LA model becomes a matter of ongoing organizational research driven by the initial study. The VNAF-LA has created a data driven smart (learning) system that allows ongoing cost data to be added to the existing database to refine the baseline results of capitation development. This approach, the baseline capitation development model, allows an organization to move away from historical cost/billing data (derived most often from Medicare/fee-for-service models of care) into the use of modeling based on demographic and cost factors that are "known" to impact utilization. It is this actual database that enables the VNAF-LA to provide care management, a focus on the client and services, as a means of cost control versus the more punitive means of cost control–utilization management. Patient care and the focus on patient needs (based on actual case experience) becomes the driving factor in managing service delivery as opposed to prospective use of controls developed on retrospective and antique billing and utilization data systems.

Network development/enrollment and marketing. Network development on the part of the sub-contractor should be viewed as capacity development and engagement in affiliations. The Visiting Nurse Association, as part of network affiliation, has begun to meet with primary care provider groups who serve HIV/AIDS patients and has started to educate these providers on the outcome of the Transprofessional Model of care through educational forums and case conference sessions. The approach taken by the VNAF-LA is one of offering insights into care management as a means of demonstrating the VNAF-LA's ability to manage both its own risk and to protect the escalating risk that is assumed by the primary provider organization. Contracting for services then becomes a matter of providing primary contractors with capitation study results and establishing competitive rates based on the case capitation approach as discussed above.

Plan licensure and certification. Much of what constitutes normal operation licensing for a home care agency sub-contractor qualifies this agency to contract with a primary health maintenance organization. There are no other conditions that must be met by the sub-contractor in providing care to HMO patients. It should be noted, however, that there are reporting requirements demanded by the primary contracting group of the sub-contractor. These requirements should be fully disclosed and negotiated as part of the initial contract.

Monitoring and quality assurance. As a sub-contractor in home care, the VNAF-LA has utilized its health research capability to mount a continuous learning process to keep informed of HMO patient utilization of services and to engage primary contractors in the use and findings from this data. The VNAF-LA views monitoring and quality assurance as products of a fee-for-service environment and utilizes the notion of a continuous quality improvement and continuous learning process as a means of being informed and staying informed with regard to service delivery and service utilization. Monitoring and quality assurance are for the most part retrospective systems of control that do not lend themselves to the managed care environment. An ongoing, continuous process of data use, analysis, and reflection is needed to improve services and to support the care decision process. To this end, patient utilization and cost data are formatted as ongoing research and have been put on-line in the VNAF-LA, made available to all levels of the organization involved in providing and managing care. Data is available on a 'real-time' basis so that patient level and service delivery level data can be accessed as needed. The key to a successful quality improvement effort directed at patient care is to have meaningful information available when it is needed as feedback to providers and administrators.

This data is then utilized by service delivery teams to inform their practices and to develop care management standards that can benefit both quality of services and cost efficiencies/effectiveness. Since the data is designed as a research/learning enterprise, outcomes of care (both clinical) and service are developed by the work teams and built into the online information system so that progress can be monitored. This type of learning system, composed of service utilization data and outcome data, then becomes a feedback system that is also capable of serving as a patient advocacy system. Outcomes especially are focused on patient identified issues. The continuous review of this data by both providers and administrators assures the patient that patient specific care issues are fed back to the whole system of care provision–those who deliver care and those to whom providers of care report.

Training and education. In a managed care environment learning is required at both the provider level and the consumer level. Learning requires that both staff members and patients be presented with information about a managed care environment. In this regard, learning takes place for staff during regular case conference sessions and in care coordination sessions (case conferences) with physicians. Patient education, while being supplemented with collateral printed material, takes place during regular home visits and during admitting visits. In a managed care environment it is critical to engage in information dissemination through routine aspects of the work day as opposed to engaging in special and infrequent (due to costs) training sessions.

Impact of VNAF-LA Organizational Restructuring on Managed Care Environment

In Fall 1997, VNAF-LA went from a private non-profit to a private for-profit organization. Several factors contributed to this, one of which was the inability of VNAF-LA to get costs low enough to be competitive in the current market. In addition, the organizational infrastructure (as is the case of many not-for-profits) allowed for the inclusion of indigent care. An example of this is that case managers would visit a patient at home whether or not they received reimbursement. While these methods may have been effective, they were not particularly efficient. VNAF-LA was purchased by Sun Healthcare Group, who subsequently reconfigured the organization. Newly titled Sun Plus Home Health examined what it could provide with the specific available dollars. Recognizing that it was no longer risk free, Sun Healthcare began extensive utilization of case management, case plans, and case planning. In addition, the organization began to look at the number of home visits and questioned whether it was necessary for RN case managers to be responsible for all home visits, whether it was possible to make contact by telephone alone, or whether it was possible for another healthcare worker, such as a physical therapist, to handle some of the activities previously handled by RN case managers. Clearly, this change enhanced the case management environment of Sun Healthcare and allowed for managed risk.

CONCLUSIONS

VNAF-LA's Transprofessional, or continuity of care, Model has demonstrated that it is possible to increase cost efficiency and increase effectiveness in meeting patient needs. Using an interdisciplinary, case-management approach (including a blending of curative and palliative services), produces a difference in the types of service providers delivering care to terminal AIDS patients as compared to the Traditional Model of care that is case managed by a nurse and is primarily focused on curative services. The project also established that a psychosocial orientation in home care is more efficient and more effective than a pure medical orientation in home care, producing lower visit and supply costs for the entire episode of care when compared to the Traditional treatment approach. The interdisciplinary nature of the model allows allied health professionals to build a complimentary case-management plan that results in less duplication of services when compared to the Traditional model. While VNAF-LA and other home care companies contracting in a managed care environment are still at some risk, using the case rate capitation approach has allowed VNAF-LA to manage their risk with a far greater benefit to the organization.

REFERENCES

Anderson, H., & MacElveen-Hoehn, P. (1988). Gay clients with AIDS: New Challenges for hospice programs. *Hospice Journal, 4* (2), 37-54.

Bulwalda, P., Kruijthoff, D. J., de Bruyn, M., & Hogewoning, A. (1994). Evaluation of a home-care/counseling AIDS programme in Kgatleng District, Botswana. *AIDS Care, 6* (2), 153-160.

Cherin, D. A., Huba, G. J., Brief, D. E., & Melchior, L. A. (1998). Evaluation of the transprofessional model of home health care for HIV/AIDS. *Home Health Care Services Quarterly, 17* (1), 55-72.

Ferrari, J. R., McCown, W., & Pantano, J. (1993). Experiencing satisfaction and stress as an AIDS care provider: The AIDS Caregiver Scale. *Evaluation & the Health Professions, 16* (3), 225-310.

Foley, F. J., Flannery, J., Grayton, D., Flintoft, R., & Cook, D. (1995). The culture of caring: AIDS palliative care: Changing the palliative paradigm. *Journal of Palliative Care, 11* (2), 19-22.

Gamliel, S., Politzer, R. M., Rivo, M. L., & Mullan, F. (1995). Managed care on the march: Will physicians meet the challenge. *Health Affairs, 14* (2), 131-142.

Gamliel, S., Singer, B., & Marconi, K. (1998). HIV Healthcare Delivery and Managed Care: Applications and Implications from the Special Projects of National Significance Program. *Home Health Care Services Quarterly, 17* (1), 101-109.

Huba, G. J., Brief, D. E., Cherin, D. A., Panter, A. T. & Melchior, L. A. (1998). A typology of service patterns in end stage AIDS care: Relationships to the transprofessional model. *Home Health Care Services Quarterly, 17* (1), 73-92.

Huba, G. J., Cherin, D. A., & Melchior, L. A. (1998). Retention of Clients in Service under Two Models of Home Health Care for HIV/AIDS. *Home Health Care Services Quarterly, 17* (3), 17-26.

Melchior, L. A., DeVeauuse, N., & Huba, G. J. (1998). Qualitative issues related to the transprofessional model of end-stage AIDS care. *Home Health Care Services Quarterly, 17* (1), 93-100.

Injection Drug Use (IDU) Related Human Immunodeficiency Virus Infection in Rural Vermont: A Comparison with Non-IDU Related Infections

Christopher Grace, MD
Karen Richardson-Nassif, PhD
Lu-Ann Rolley
Deborah Kutzko, FNP
Kemper Alston, MD
Marybeth Ramundo, MD

SUMMARY. The epidemic of HIV infection is spreading into rural areas of the United States. Injection drug use (IDU) is contributing to this spread in a manner similar to that of larger urban areas. The pur-

Christopher Grace, Deborah Kutzko, Kemper Alston, and Marybeth Ramundo are affiliated with the Department of Medicine, University of Vermont, Burlington, VT. Karen Richardson-Nassif and Lu-Ann Rolley are affiliated with the Department of Family Practice, University of Vermont, Burlington, VT.

Address correspondence to: Christopher Grace, MD, Associate Professor of Medicine, University of Vermont, Fletcher Allen Health Care, Brown 325, Burlington, VT 05401.

This work was supported in part by the Health Resources and Services Administration (HRSA), HIV/AIDS Bureau (HAB), Special Projects of National Significance (SPNS) Grant No. 5 U90 HA 00026-05. This publication's contents are solely the responsibility of the authors and do not necessarily represent the official view of the funding agency.

[Haworth co-indexing entry note]: "Injection Drug Use (IDU) Related Human Immunodeficiency Virus Infection in Rural Vermont: A Comparison with Non-IDU Related Infections." Grace, Christopher et al. Co-published simultaneously in *Drugs & Society* (The Haworth Press, Inc.) Vol. 16, No. 1/2, 2000, pp. 223-235; and: *Evaluating HIV/AIDS Treatment Programs: Innovative Methods and Findings* (ed: G. J. Huba et al.) The Haworth Press, Inc., 2000, pp. 223-235. Single or multiple copies of this article are available for a fee from The Haworth Document Delivery Service [1-800-342-9678, 9:00 a.m. - 5:00 p.m. (EST). E-mail address: getinfo@haworthpressinc.com].

223

pose of this paper is to assess the extent that IDU contributes to the HIV epidemic in Vermont and to compare this group of patients to others infected by HIV by non-IDU means. Twenty-three percent of 119 HIV-positive patients attending rural clinics in Vermont identified IDU as the most likely route of their HIV infection. Another 25% were infected by heterosexual contact with someone at risk for HIV. The majority of patients reported that they became infected with HIV outside of Vermont. Over 40% of IDU patients were first diagnosed with HIV after moving to Vermont. Proportionately more women and minorities were HIV infected by IDU when compared to men and white non-Hispanic patients. The great majority of IDUs were unemployed and depended on welfare or disability for financial support. All IDUs had either Medicaid or Medicare. Most IDU patients had advanced HIV infection upon presentation, with 56% having AIDS and 74% having CD4 counts less than 500 cells/mm. IDU is having a large impact on the HIV epidemic in Vermont both medically and economically and is contributing to the growing epidemic in rural America. *[Article copies available for a fee from The Haworth Document Delivery Service: 1-800-342-9678. E-mail address: <getinfo@haworthpressinc.com> Website: <http://www.HaworthPress.com>]*

KEYWORDS. Injection drug use, rural, HIV/AIDS

INTRODUCTION

The epidemics of the Acquired Immune Deficiency Syndrome (AIDS) and injection drug use (IDU) have traditionally been considered a phenomenon of large metropolitan areas, especially in the Northeast United States (Allen, 1992). Both epidemics, however, have spread rapidly into rural areas of the United States (Lam & Liu, 1994). From 1991 to 1992 non-metropolitan areas' AIDS cases increased 9.4% compared to 3.1% in metropolitan areas (Berry, 1993). The rate of AIDS among men who have sex with men (MSM) increased disproportionately in rural as compared to urban areas (Centers for Disease Control and Prevention, 1995). This increase may be related not only to patients infected and diagnosed in rural areas but also to migration of Human Immunodeficiency Virus (HIV) infected persons from urban to rural settings (Fordycee, Thomas, & Shum, 1997; Cohen, Klein, Mohr, van der Horst, & Weber, 1994).

IDU has played a major role in the AIDS pandemic. Since the first IDU related case report in 1981 in New York City, IDU has become an increasingly prevalent means of transmission of HIV in the United States, Europe and developing countries. From the late 1980s to early 1990s, there was a 136% increase in IDU related AIDS infections (Quinn, 1995). Thirty-three percent of AIDS infections in the U.S. can be attributed to IDU (Alcabes & Freidland,

1995). This number includes 24% of AIDS patients whose risk was IDU, as well as 4% of patients whose only risk was unprotected intercourse with an injection drug user and 5% of patients who had both IDU and sexual risk behaviors (Pickens, Battljes, Svikis, & Gupman, 1993). The number of AIDS cases attributable to IDU is the same in large metropolitan statistical areas (MSA) as it is in non-MSA areas (Steel, Fleming, & Needle, 1993).

Vermont is one of the most rural states in the nation. It has a population of 588,654 persons (1996) living within 9,615 square miles in northern New England. The largest city, Burlington, in the northwestern quadrant of the state, has a population of 50,000 persons. Sixty-eight percent of the state population lives in towns of less than 2,500. Ninety-eight percent of the population is White Non-Hispanic, 0.4% African American, 0.7% Asian, 0.6% Hispanic, and 0.3% Native American.

The first case of AIDS was reported in Vermont in 1982. As of September 1998, there were 340 reported cases of AIDS in the state. Eighty-eight percent of the reported patients are White Non-Hispanic, 7% African American, and 4% Hispanic. Men who have sex with men account for 59% of the cases, IDU for 19%, and MSM/IDU for 5%. Heterosexual transmission accounts for 7%, while blood products caused 5%. No known cause of transmission is reported by 5%. Prior to 1994, women made up only 8% of AIDS cases. During 1994-1995, women comprised 15% of cases. Fifty-four percent of these women were exposed heterosexually, 43% by injection drug use and 4% by blood transfusion. HIV infection is not reportable in Vermont. Therefore, the prevalence of HIV infection in the state is unknown. The Vermont Department of Health (VDH) estimates there are between 335-430 people living with HIV in Vermont. It is estimated that 50-60% of new infections will be MSM, 24-41% IDU, 9-22% people of color, and up to 26% women (Vermont, 1998).

There are currently four HIV specialty clinics in the state. The first, established in Burlington in 1987, is located in the most populous area in the state. The other three clinics opened during the last four years with support from the Special Projects of National Significance (SPNS) of the Health Resources Service Administration (HRSA). The purpose of the SPNS Vermont project was to develop HIV specialty clinics that: provide state-of-the-art HIV healthcare in rural areas of Vermont; reduce barriers interfering with people receiving their healthcare in their own communities; and establish a collaborative care and teaching network with regional providers. Each of the three rural clinics is located in a quadrant of the state, which previously did not have regional HIV specialty care. The clinics, housed in regional hospitals, are staffed by an infectious disease specialist who travels to the clinic once per month, a nurse practitioner, a social worker and a representative from regional AIDS service organizations. Philosophically, the Vermont model of

HIV care delivery shifts the emphasis of care to the HIV specialist who leads a team of providers who render both primary and HIV specialty care. Patients in rural areas are able to receive complete medical care, psychosocial support and drug and alcohol assessment and referral (Grace, Soons, Kutzko, Alston, & Ramundo, in press). The four Vermont clinics provide care to the vast majority of HIV infected persons in the state.

An evaluation team coordinates project data collection and evaluation. Patient data are collected at the initial visit and at each follow-up visit to the physician or nurse practitioner as well as at social worker visits. Data collected includes patient demographics, medical insurance, financial support, healthcare utilization, HIV transmission risks and patient migration patterns, medical care including prophylaxis and antiretroviral therapy, psychosocial issues, and access and barriers to care. Patients also complete satisfaction and quality of life questionnaires yearly. These data serve to address how well the program has met its goals of: (a) providing HIV care in rural areas of the state including antiretroviral therapy, opportunistic infection prophylaxis, appropriate screening tests and immunizations; and (b) psychosocial assessment and support. Additionally, the data assist in defining the epidemiology of the HIV epidemic in rural Vermont.

Much of the rural IDU-related HIV infection has been documented in the Southeastern U.S.A. especially among African American women (Whyte & Carr, 1992). The purpose of this study is to assess the extent that IDU contributes to the HIV epidemic in this rural area of the northeastern United States and the effects on healthcare delivery in Vermont.

METHODS

Participants

From October 1994 through October 1998, 126 patients have received care at one of the three SPNS supported clinics. This represents 48% of the 261 new patients cared for in one of the four HIV specialty clinics in Vermont during this time period. The other 135 patients received care in the Burlington clinic and are not included in this analysis. One hundred and nineteen of these 126 patients (94%) signed consent and represent the data presented.

Measures

All patients receiving care at the three SPNS supported rural specialty clinics were asked to complete an 11 page initial questionnaire during their first clinic visit. This questionnaire included information regarding patient demographics, access and barriers to care, patient migration, HIV medical history, medications, laboratory, and psychosocial issues.

Procedures

All participating patients signed a consent form approved by the University of Vermont Institutional Review Board. The clinic nurse practitioner or physician administered the questionnaire. Patient data are grouped by HIV transmission mode. Group I includes patients who reported HIV transmission as either IDU or IDU/MSM. Group II included patients who reported their means of HIV transmission either as MSM, heterosexual contact with a person at risk, blood product recipient, or unknown.

Statistical Analysis

Chi-square analysis was performed to detect differences between Groups I and II with independent samples and t-test analysis for the continuous age variable.

RESULTS

The HIV transmission risk for 27 patients (23%) was IDU or IDU/MSM (Group I). Ninety-two patients (77%) were not infected directly by injection drug use (Group II). Group II included MSM 59 (64%), heterosexual contact with someone at risk 30 (33%), unknown risk 9 (10%), and blood product related 1 (1%). Group II comes to greater than 100% because patients were able to select more than one risk factor (99 responses from the 92 patients). Ages were similar between the two groups (IDU–39 years, range 26-51; non-IDU–40 years, range 18-62). Minority groups (Hispanic, African American, American Indian/Alaskan native) were more frequently infected by IDU (22%) than non-IDU (13%). Proportionally more women (30%) were infected by IDU than men (21%) were. Three (43%) of the seven IDU infected women were non-white as compared to two (6%) of the 16 non-IDU infected women. However, due to the small numbers these differences were not statistically significant.

Data illustrating employment status and means of financial support are shown in Table 1. There were incomplete data from 14 of the non-IDU group regarding employment status and one from the IDU group. Three (12 percent) of the IDU infected patients were employed as compared to 39 (42 percent) of the non-IDU patients, $p = .003$. For those who were unemployed, the rates of various distributions of financial support are also illustrated in Table 1. The majority of unemployed members from both groups were either on disability or welfare.

Figure 1 illustrates the geographic location where patients were infected and diagnosed with HIV. The majority of IDUs and non-IDUs felt they were infected outside the state of Vermont, although a greater percentage of IDU patients were infected outside of Vermont than non-IDU patients (Group I, 96% vs. Group II, 72%, $p = .015$). Large minorities of both groups (44% for IDU and 42% for non-IDU) were first diagnosed with HIV after moving to Vermont.

TABLE 1. Employment Status and Means of Support: IDU vs. Non-IDU

	IDU Number (%)	Non-IDU Number (%)	p Value
Total patients	27	92	
Employed (yes)	3 (12)	39 (42)	0.003
Financial support			
If not employed (*);			
Number	22	53	
Disability	18 (82)	32 (60)	NS
Welfare	4 (18)	9 (17)	NS
Family, none, other	3 (15)	18 (33)	NS

Note. IDU = HIV infected by injection drug use; Non-IDU = HIV infected sexually, blood products or unknown. NS = not statistically significant. (*) = 24 IDU patients were unemployed, 2 had missing data. There were 25 responses from the 22 IDU patients and 59 responses from the 53 non-IDU patients since patients could select more than one category.

Most patients from either group had advanced HIV infection when they entered the clinic program. Fifty-six percent of the IDU group as compared to 35% of the non-IDU group had AIDS at the time of their initial visit. Figure 2 illustrates the CD4 count at the initial visit. Greater than 70% of both groups had CD4 counts less than 500 cells/mm of blood.

Figure 3 illustrates the type of medical insurance held by patients of the clinics. Several patients from both groups had more than one type of insurance accounting for the greater than 100% response rate. The majority of patients had either Medicaid or Medicare. Seven percent of the IDU patients had private insurance which was significantly different from 30% of non-IDU patients ($p = .017$). A small minority (11% of IDU vs. 20% non-IDU) of both groups had no health insurance. Significantly more IDU patients had Medicaid than non-IDU patients ($p = .001$). There was no difference between the groups with respect to Medicare coverage.

DISCUSSION

Injection drug use has contributed to HIV transmission in up to 36% of AIDS cases reported to the Centers for Disease Control and Prevention as of 1996 (Paone, Des Jarlais, Clark, Shi, Kim, & Purchase, 1997). Women and

FIGURE 1. State of HIV Infection and Diagnosis: IDU (*n* = 24) vs. Non-IDU (*n* = 72)

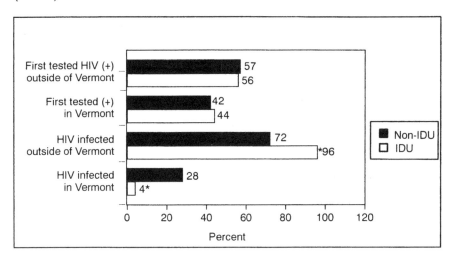

Note *p* = .015

FIGURE 2. CD4 Counts at Initial Visit to Vermont Rural Clinic: IDU (*n* = 25) vs. Non-IDU (*n* = 81)

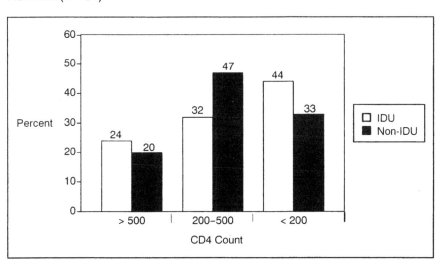

FIGURE 3. Type of Medical Insurance: IDU vs. Non-IDU

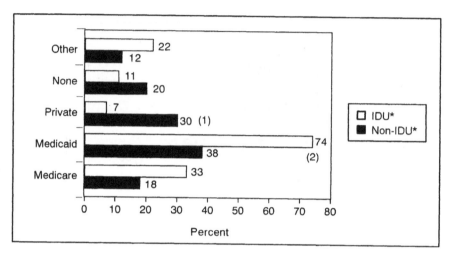

*Note   *IDU Infected: 40 responses from 27 patients*
Non-IDU Infected: 113 responses from 92 patients
(1) p = .015
(2) p = .001

minorities are disproportionately affected by this transmission mode with IDU accounting for 36% of AIDS transmission in women, especially women of color (Centers for Disease Control and Prevention, 1996). Traditionally felt to be a scourge of large cities, IDU has now been shown to be a major means of HIV transmission in rural areas of this country as well (Graham, Forrester, Wysong, Rosenthal, & James, 1995). The first wave of HIV infection in rural areas among gay men is now being augmented by a second wave. This second wave, affecting women, minorities, migrant workers, and adolescents disproportionately, is due in large part to IDU, crack cocaine use, and exchanging sex for drugs (Lam & Liu, 1994). This is especially true in the Southeastern United States (Graham et al., 1995). Whyte and Carr (1992) showed that of 142 women with AIDS in rural areas of Georgia, 76% were African American and 71% of infections were related directly or indirectly to IDU. Cohen et al. (1994) documented similar patterns in North Carolina. Wooten (1989) in rural California has described a different epidemiology. In rural California the epidemic still disproportionately affects gay white men although IDU and IDU plus MSM accounted for 24.2% of infections in rural California, while women and minorities accounted for 8.1% of AIDS patients.

The evaluation of this SPNS project allowed not only an assessment of the goals and objectives of the Vermont model but also provided an opportunity to examine the epidemiology of HIV in this rural patient population. Program evaluation data is essential to measure and track existing patient needs as well as to help plan future care needs. It will be important for other rural HIV healthcare programs to collect information on transmission risk, employment, health insurance and degree of illness to better assess the extent that IDU is having on HIV service delivery in rural areas of the country. Additionally issues especially pertinent to rural areas including transportation needs, confidentiality in small towns and extent of psychosocial support and substance abuse counseling and care will need to be studied for this patient population. Collection of health finance data will be important in order to measure the effect of IDU-related HIV illness on resource utilization. This will be true not only for rural states such as Vermont, but also for rural areas of states with large metropolitan areas such as New York and California.

The evaluation of this SPNS model emphasized the large impact that IDU is having on the HIV epidemic in Vermont. Using data evaluation processes in healthcare programs will help states, hospitals and healthcare service providers predict additional services that will be required to meet the changing needs of the patient population. For example, the large number of IDU infected persons raises concerns about the effect co-infection with hepatitis C virus (HCV) may have on IDU infected patients in rural areas.

Twenty-three percent of the patients being cared for in rural Vermont were infected by IDU. Thirty of the 119 patients were infected heterosexually, further increasing the potential effects of IDU in this population. Sexual contact with an injection drug user has accounted for most cases of heterosexually acquired AIDS in the United States (Neal, Fleming, Green, & Ward, 1997). These numbers are similar to those reviewed by Steel et al. (1993) who found that approximately 50% of persons from large MSAs, small MSAs and non-MSAs had HIV infection attributable directly or indirectly to IDU. The impact that IDU has had on the HIV epidemic in this rural state is as extensive as it has been in other rural states (Steel & Haverkos, 1992). The Vermont Department of Health (1998) attributed IDU or MSM/IDU to 24% of risk transmission throughout the state, which is very similar to the risk stratification in the rural clinics. Only 7% of patients with AIDS, reported to the Vermont Department of Health, attributed heterosexual contact with a person at risk as the means of transmission. This is similar to the 8.4%-10.4% heterosexual transmission risk in the Midwest and western parts of the U.S. (Neal et al., 1997) though less than in rural Vermont (25%). If the partner at risk was an IDU then the influence of IDU may be greater in the rural areas of Vermont than in the more metropolitan areas of the state.

The epidemiology of the epidemic in Vermont is similar with epidemiological patterns in both the southeast United States and in California. Proportionately more women are infected by IDU directly than non-IDU (30% vs. 21%). The same is true of minority patients (22% vs. 13%). This is especially evident when it is recognized that less than 3% of Vermont residents are African American, Hispanic, Asian, or Native American, while 15% of the clinic patients are minorities. Forty-three percent of women infected by IDU are minorities as compared to 6% of women infected by non-IDU means.

Migration of IDU infected persons into rural areas has accounted for a growing part of the rural epidemic (Fordycee et al., 1997; Cohen et al., 1994). Rumley, Shappley, Waivers et al. (1992) from North Carolina found that 55% of patients with AIDS and 40% of patients with HIV had migrated into the state. Most patients seeking care in rural Vermont felt they were infected with HIV outside the state, with high rates for IDU (96%) and non-IDU (72%) making migration a vital aspect of the epidemic in this state. Despite the majority of patients being infected outside of Vermont, a large minority, 44% for IDU and 42% for non-IDU, were first diagnosed with HIV after coming to Vermont. *It needs to be recognized that the HIV/AIDS epidemic in rural America consists of persons infected with HIV while living in a rural area and also patients moving to rural areas from urban centers who are already infected. This migratory group of patients increases demand for services in rural areas including medical care, financial assistance and community-based case management. These issues are particularly of concern when caring for IDU patients. The complex medical care these patients require will need to be furnished by HIV expert and experienced providers. The Vermont model addresses this issue by placing experienced providers in rural areas of the state. Additionally there is a real concern that the migration of infected persons will increase in state HIV transmission, further worsening the epidemic in rural areas.*

The majority of both IDU and non-IDU patients were unemployed and depended on disability or welfare for financial support. Significantly more IDU were unemployed (88%) than non-IDU. These numbers are similar to unemployment rates among IDU in New York City (78%) and larger than the percentage of unemployed IDU in Miami or Houston (45%) (Pickens et al., 1993). All IDU had either Medicaid or Medicare for health insurance as compared to about only half of non-IDU. These findings may reinforce the findings of Rumley et al. (1992) who felt the large migration of HIV infected patients to rural North Carolina was due to IDU seeking more social supports. Identification of these trends will help federal and state agencies plan for additional services.

Upon initial evaluation at the clinics, 56% of the IDU and 35% of the non-IDU had AIDS. This is higher than the average 28% initial AIDS diagnosis found in other states in the South, Midwest and West (Centers for Disease Control and Prevention, 1998). Over 70% of both groups had CD4 counts less than 500 cells/mm. This advanced level of infection in the majority of patients suggests that patients are not accessing care early in their illness leaving them susceptible to opportunistic infections and less likely to have prolonged responses to antiretroviral therapy. *This may also lead to increased emergency department visits and hospitalizations, increasing morbidity and possibly mortality for patients and costs for the healthcare system. This IDU infected patient population further emphasizes the need to remove barriers to accessing medical care in rural areas. Although the Vermont model of care has removed many barriers to accessing care, greater efforts at outreach aimed at the growing number of IDU infected patients are greatly needed.*

Injection drug use is playing a significant role in the HIV epidemic in Vermont. Patients are being infected out of state, migrating to Vermont and presenting to care with advanced levels of illness. High unemployment and inadequate insurance in this patient group will increase economic risk to health providers and the state social welfare programs. Co-morbid conditions in as many as 50-80% of IDUs, including mental illness, chronic liver disease and complex psychosocial problems, add to the complexity of care (Ferrando, Wall, Batki, & Sorenson, 1996). As the number of people living with HIV move to and seek care in this state, greater numbers of patients will need social services including housing, financial support, transportation, government supported health insurance, drug and alcohol treatment programs, HIV and IDU risk reduction intervention and clinic coordinated psychosocial support. Active drug use has been associated with poor compliance to medications raising concerns of viral resistance in the patient and transmission of resistant HIV to others (Sherer, 1998). HIV infected injection drug users may not be receiving optimal care with as many as 86% not receiving triple combination therapy in Baltimore (Celentano, Vlahov, Cohn, Shadle, Obasanjo, & Moore, 1998) and only 40% receiving any antiretroviral drugs in British Columbia despite the free cost of therapy (Strathdee, Palepu, Cornelisse, Yip, O'Shaughnessy, Montaner et al., 1998). Greater efforts at outreach, HIV testing, drug abuse counseling and HIV medical care are needed for this group of people in urban and rural areas alike. Program evaluation can help organize patient data, measure trends and highlight changes in patient populations served by healthcare providers. By monitoring patient demographics, health and utilized services, healthcare institutions can better meet current needs and help predict future obligations.

REFERENCES

Alcabes, P., & Freidland, F. (1995). Injection drug use and human immunodeficiency virus infection. *Clinical Infectious Diseases, 20,* 1467-1479.

Allen, D. A. (1992). HIV infection in intravenous drug users entering drug treatment, United States, 1988 to 1989. *American Journal of Public Health, 82,* 541-546.

Berry, D. E. (1993). The emerging epidemiology of rural AIDS. *Journal of Rural Health, 9*, (4), 193-304.

Celentano, D. D., Vlahov, D., Cohn, S., Shadle, V. M., Obasanjo, O., & Moore, R. D. (1998). Self-reporting antiretroviral therapy in injection drug users. *JAMA, 280,* 544-546.

Centers for Disease Control and Prevention. (1998). Diagnosis and reporting of HIV and AIDS in states with integrated HIV and AIDS surveillance–United States, January 1994-June 1997. *Morbidity and Mortality Weekly Report, 47* (15), 309-314.

Centers for Disease Control and Prevention. (1996). *HIV/AIDS Surveillance Report, 8* (1) (Midyear Edition). Atlanta.

Centers for Disease Control and Prevention. (1995). Update; trends in AIDS among men who have sex with men–United States. 1989-1994. *Morbidity and Mortality Weekly Report, 44* (21), 401-404.

Cohen, S. E., Klein, J. D., Mohr, J. E., van der Horst, C. M., & Weber, D. J. (1994). The geography of AIDS: Patterns of urban and rural migration. *Southern Medical Journal, 87,* 599-606.

Ferrando, S. J., Wall, T. L., Batki, S. L. & Sorenson, J. L. (1996). Psychiatric morbidity, illicit drug use and adherence to zidovudine (AZT) among injection drug users with HIV disease. *American Journal of Drug and Alcohol Abuse, 22,* 475-487.

Fordycee, E. J., Thomas, P., & Shum, R. (1997). Evidence of an increasing AIDS burden in rural America. *Statistical Bulletin, 78,* 2-9.

Grace, C., Soons, K., Kutzko, D., Alston, W., & Ramundo, M. (in press). Service delivery for patients with human immunodeficiency virus in a rural state; the Vermont model. *AIDS Patient Care and STDs.*

Graham, R. P., Forrester, M. L., Wysong, J. A., Rosenthal, T. C., & James, P. A. (1995). HIV/AIDS in the rural United States: Epidemiology and health services delivery. *Medical Care Research and Review, 52,* 435-452.

Lam, N. S., & Liu, K. B. (1994). Spread of AIDS into rural America. *Journal of Acquired Immune Deficiency Syndromes, 7,* 485-490.

Neal, J. L., Fleming, P. L., Green, T. A., & Ward, J. W. (1997). Trends in heterosexually acquired AIDS in the United States, 1988 through 1995. *Journal of Acquired Immune Deficiency Syndromes. 14,* 465-474.

Pickens, R. W., Battjes, R., Svikis, D. S., & Gupman, A. E. (1993). Substance abuse risk factors for HIV infection. *Psychiatric Clinics of North America, 16,* 119-125.

Paone, D., Des Jarlais, D., Clark, J., Shi, Q., Krim, M., & Purchase, D. (1997). Syringe exchange programs–United States, 1996. *Morbidity and Mortality Weekly Report, 46,* 565-568.

Quinn, T. C. (1995). The epidemiology of the acquired immunodeficiency syndrome in the 1990's. *Emergency Medicine Clinics of North America, 13,* 1-25.

Rumley, R. L., Shappley, N. C., Waivers, L. E. et al. (1992). The impact of HIV patient migration to rural areas. *AIDS Patient Care and STDs, 6,* 225-228.

Sherer, R. (1998). Adherence and antiretroviral therapy in injection drug users. *JAMA, 280,* 567-568.

Steel, E., & Haverkos, H. W. (1992). AIDS and drug use in rural America. *Journal of Rural Health, 8,* 70-73.

Steel, M., Fleming, P., & Needle, R. (1993). HIV rates of injection drug users in less-populated areas. *American Journal of Public Health, 83,* 286-287.

Strathdee, S. A., Palepu, A., Cornelisse, P. G. A., Yip, B., O'Shaughnessy, O. B. C., Montaner, J. G., Schechter, M. T., & Hogg, R. S. (1998). Barriers to use of free antiretroviral therapy in injection drug users. *JAMA, 280,* 547-549.

Vermont Department of Health. (1998). *Vermont AIDS Report.* AIDS Program. Burlington, Vermont.

Whyte, B. M., & Carr, J. C. (1992). Comparison of AIDS in women in rural and urban Georgia. *Southern Medical Journal, 85,* 571-578.

Wooten, D. B. (1989). AIDS in rural California. *Human Services in Rural Environment, 13,* 30-33.

Evaluation
of Status and Progression of HIV Disease: Use of a Computerized Medical Module

Robert L. Brunner, PhD
Trudy A. Larson, MD
G. J. Huba, PhD
Lisa A. Melchior, PhD
Barbara J. Scott, RD, MPH

SUMMARY. The Northern Nevada HOPES (HIV Outpatient Program, Education, and Services) Clinic provides comprehensive and consultative care to persons living with HIV/AIDS in Reno, Nevada. As a method of tracking clinical data for evaluation purposes, a computer database was designed and implemented in the clinic setting. Analysis of these data permitted an exploration of the relations among client behaviors such as substance abuse and clinical markers of HIV disease progression. Substance abuse was found to be related to a number of indi-

Robert L. Brunner, Trudy A. Larson, and Barbara J. Scott are affiliated with the University of Nevada School of Medicine, Reno, NV. G. J. Huba and Lisa A. Melchior are affiliated with The Measurement Group, Culver City, CA.

Address correspondence to: Robert L. Brunner, PhD, Nutrition Education and Research Program, University of Nevada School of Medicine, Mailstop 153, Reno, NV 89557-0046 (E-mail: brunner@scs.unr.edu).

This work was supported in part by the Health Resources and Services Administration (HRSA), HIV/AIDS Bureau (HAB), Special Projects of National Significance (SPNS) Grant No. 5 U90 HA 00038-05. This publication's contents are solely the responsibility of the authors and do not necessarily represent the official view of the funding agency.

[Haworth co-indexing entry note]: "Evaluation of Status and Progression of HIV Disease: Use of a Computerized Medical Module." Brunner, Robert L. et al. Co-published simultaneously in *Drugs & Society* (The Haworth Press, Inc.) Vol. 16, No. 1/2, 2000, pp. 237-249; and: *Evaluating HIV/AIDS Treatment Programs: Innovative Methods and Findings* (ed: G. J. Huba et al.) The Haworth Press, Inc., 2000, pp. 237-249. Single or multiple copies of this article are available for a fee from The Haworth Document Delivery Service [1-800-342-9678, 9:00 a.m. - 5:00 p.m. (EST). E-mail address: getinfo@haworthpressinc.com].

cators of impaired health. The computerized medical data module was found to be a useful tool for evaluation and quality assurance purposes and permitted the quantification of substance abuse behaviors in the clinic population. *[Article copies available for a fee from The Haworth Document Delivery Service: 1-800-342-9678. E-mail address: <getinfo@haworthpress inc.com> Website: <http://www.HaworthPress.com>]*

KEYWORDS. HIV/AIDS, data, comprehensive healthcare

INTRODUCTION

The Northern Nevada HOPES (HIV Outpatient Program, Education and Services) Clinic provides comprehensive and consultative care to HIV-positive clients coming from a wide demographic spectrum and with a range of disease states. Overall, the clinic demographics demonstrate that substance abuse; past or present is a growing issue. This clinic has an active (seen in the last year) patient population of 180. At the start of the work presented here, the clinic staff consisted of six physicians (all part-time), two registered nurses, an administrative nurse, receptionist and pharmacist (part-time). The organization of the clinic has since changed, as has the staff composition with the addition of a social worker and outreach nurse.

Beginning in 1995, patients in the clinic were offered nutrition services as part of the "Early Nutrition Intervention in HIV/AIDS" project. This project, funded as a Special Project of National Significance, was designed to test the benefits of nutrition intervention as a means of preventing weight loss and wasting in HIV disease (Scott, Larson, Brunner, Navarro, & Mathes, 1999). The program was introduced to potential participants as a study intended to learn how to prevent weight loss and wasting by prospective assessment of nutritional status and by provision of ongoing personal nutrition counseling over the course of five years.

To assess the key outcome measures for the project of overall health and medical status, a database was constructed by retrospective review of participants' medical charts from the HOPES clinic using a computerized medical module to guide the data collection and entry.

Two long-term goals of creating the medical database were to (1) compare the health and disease status of patients who received nutrition services to those who did not; and (2) compare patient health, disease and quality of life prior to and after starting nutrition services. The information presented here is derived from an interim analysis, which describes the medical status of patients in a community HIV clinic who participated in the nutrition project. The influence of substance use on medical outcomes is also evaluated. In addition, this paper illustrates how a computerized data tool can be used to evaluate quality of care in terms of consistency, completeness, follow-up, and documentation.

METHODS

Participants

Chart reviews were completed for 38 people (32 men and 6 women; mean age = 35 years) who had an average of 9.6 (min = 1; max = 34) visits to the clinic between 1995 when the chart reviews began and the end of 1997 when they were completed. A total number of 365 clinic visits were reviewed. While most of these participants had advanced or long standing HIV disease, the length of time since infection was not known.

Alcohol, Drug and Tobacco Use

Participants completed a questionnaire in which they reported past or current tobacco, illicit drug and injection drug use and "problems" with alcohol. Three participants did not respond to one or more items. Among men, 13 reported "never" using tobacco, seven "past" use and 11 "current" use. Women's tobacco use was similar: never (n = 2), past (n =1) and current (n = 3). Only one man reported current alcohol problems, and 20 reported no history, while 11 reported a history of problems in the past. The group of women was evenly split between never having alcohol problems and a past history of problems. Among men, 13 reported never using illicit drugs, 13 had past use and four were currently using. None of the women reported current drug use, three reported never using and two reported past use. No one reported current injection drug use, but nine men and one woman reported past use with the remaining participants reporting no illicit drug related needle experiences.

Data Management

The data from the medical charts were recorded in a custom designed, computerized application developed by The Measurement Group. This software application included data fields for basic patient information, visits to outside healthcare providers, referrals made, symptoms, diseases (by history and current), laboratory results, Karnofsky ratings, and current medicines and supplements.

The software application for data entry was designed with an array of entry field types (multiple choice, yes-no, text) depending on the particular information being gathered. Diseases, symptoms, outside healthcare visits and referrals that were specifically reported by the registered nurse, physicians' assistant or physician in the clinical notes for the visit were entered. Multiple choice options included:

- various healthcare specialists (in the section concerned with outside referrals);
- six HIV-related symptoms (weight loss > 10%, night sweats, diarrhea > 1 month, shingles, peripheral neuropathy, and mucosal candidiasis) either by history or as a current complaint;
- medical conditions accompanying HIV (tuberculosis, abnormal Pap, sexually transmitted disease, pregnancy, dementia, and others);
- opportunistic infections either by history or as current conditions (Centers for Disease Control and Prevention, 1992); and
- common health problems associated with HIV (drug toxicity/side effects, fatigue, chronic pain, fever, nausea, vomiting, poor appetite, upper respiratory infection, flu, insomnia, rash, headache, and heartburn).

The data that were entered directly (without multiple choice options) included medications prescribed and laboratory results. Other symptoms and diseases not included as multiple choice options were entered using ICD-9 codes.

RESULTS

Medical Data Findings

Table 1 shows the frequency and percentage, in this sample, of those common HIV-related health problems that were provided as specific options in the data entry software. Night sweats were the most frequently reported symptom and the only symptom of the common HIV-related health problems reported for nearly one-half of the patients. Diarrhea was next most common and was reported in about one-third of patients. Over the three-year period, episodes of night sweats and diarrhea were reported two or three times for 56% and 50% of patients, respectively. However, for 12% and 20% of patients, night sweats and diarrhea, respectively, were reported only once. Nineteen percent of patients with night sweats and 40% of patients with diarrhea had occurrences five or more times over the three-year period. An examination of consecutive visits at which night sweats and diarrhea were reported indicated that for most patients these were not found at consecutive visits. "Isolated" or "recurrent" rather than "continuous" appear to be the most apt descriptions of the pattern of occurrence of diarrhea and night sweats. Patients with common HIV associated medical conditions that were provided as specific options in the software program (sexually transmitted diseases, dementia, tuberculosis, pregnancy, abnormal Pap) were most likely to report having had sexually transmitted diseases (34.5%). Only two patients reported having a positive PPD indicative of tuberculosis exposure, and no cases of dementia or abnormal Paps were reported. In general, opportunistic infections (OI) were rarely noted. The most common OI listed was candida of bronchi, lungs, etc., with 23.7% of patients having documentation of this condition. Herpes infections were next most common at 13.2%. Other OIs were rarely reported and included three patients with pneumocystis carinii pneumonia (7.9%) and one patient each with mycobacterium avium complex and cryptococcosis. The only AIDS defining conditions reported were wasting syndrome and Kaposi's Sarcoma in one patient each.

Table 2 shows the frequency of other common health conditions, not specifically related to HIV but common in clinical practice, that were specific options in the data entry software. These issues were addressed in clinic visits that were both regular (for routine follow-up) and acute (for illness), and the high rates of reporting common conditions such as fatigue (65.8%), headache (57.9%) and rash (47.4%) highlight the many non-specific, less serious symptoms that require intervention. Some of these conditions may be related to medication side effects or to HIV disease itself, but just as commonly may be the manifestations of increasing age and complaints seen in most primary care offices.

Many diseases or conditions not specifically offered as options in the data entry software were reported in clinical notes during visits. These were entered using ICD-9 codes and are shown in Table 3. The most frequently reported of these medical problems was numbness (which also included peripheral neuropathy when specified), stiff neck, diarrhea < 1 month, chills and shortness of breath. Reported conditions mix both non-specific complaints with more HIV-related issues and other chronic conditions. The presence of neuropathy (if defined as numbness) in 50% of patients contrasts with diagnosis of peripheral neuropathy (10.5%) as a stand alone diagnosis (Table

TABLE 1. Number of Patients with HIV-Related Symptoms (*N* = 38)

Problem	By History	Current	Percent Overlap*
Night Sweats	18 (47.4%)	19 (50.0%)	100%
Diarrhea (> 1 month)	12 (31.6%)	10 (26.3%)	90%
Shingles	8 (21.0%)	2 (5.3%)	100%
Peripheral Neuropathy	3 (7.9%)	4 (10.5%)	100%
Weight Loss ≥ 10 lb.	3 (7.9%)	3 (7.9%)	66%

Note. *Patients reporting symptoms both by history and currently.

TABLE 2. Number of Patients with Other Common Health Conditions

Medical Condition	Number (%)
Fatigue	28 (65.8%)
Headache	22 (57.9%)
Rash	18 (47.4%)
Nausea	15 (39.5%)
Fever	14 (36.9%)
Poor Appetite	11 (28.9%)
Drug toxicity/Side effects	10 (26.3%)
URI/Cold/Flu	9 (23.7%)
Heartburn	6 (15.8%)
Vomiting	6 (15.8%)
Chronic pain	4 (10.5%)
Insomnia	3 (7.9%)

1) and more accurately reflects the morbidity experienced by the patient. In another comparison, chronic pain per se was identified in the clinic note and was therefore entered as a specific common condition (using the multiple choice option) for four patients. In contrast, limb and abdominal pain, not specifically identified as chronic in the clinic note but perhaps experienced as episodic, was reported by a total of 11 patients and was entered using the ICD-9 codes. This example highlights the usefulness of using specific ICD-9 coding in identifying issues that need to be addressed with patients on a more frequent basis.

HIV Severity and Medical Symptoms

It was of interest to examine the statistical relationship between the number of symptoms reported per visit and indications of HIV severity. The mean viral load, CD4 count, CD4 percent (Table 4), and the mean number of symptoms per clinic contact were computed for each year (1995-1997). Correlation coefficients were computed among these variables by year. Only

TABLE 3. Number of Patients with Other Common Health Conditions from ICD-9 Codes

Medical Condition	Number of Patients
Peripheral neuropathy (numbness)	19
Diarrhea	13
Cough	11
Chills/Generalized pain	8
Shortness of breath	7
Pain in limb	7
Sore throat	7
Blurred vision	7
Drug or tobacco dependence	7
Malaise	6
Stiff neck	6
Dermatitis	6
Depression	5
Tachycardia, palpitations	5
Sinusitis	5
Lymphadenopathy	4
Abdominal pain	4
Other diseases of the nasal cavity and sinuses	4
Allergy (allergic rhinitis)	2

CD4 and CD4 percent were significantly correlated ($r = .81, p < .01$). Symptom number increased as CD4 decreased but not significantly ($r = -0.19$). The viral load measurements had an immense range, and neither a log nor square root transformation of these data impacted the relationship with symptom frequency. Surprisingly, the relationship between viral load and symptom number was not in the predicted direction with an inverse and non-significant correlation.

TABLE 4. Number and Percent of CD4 Cells and Viral Load by Year

Measure (mean & standard deviation)	Year		
	1995	1996	1997
CD4 Count	243.7 (193.9)	270.5 (209.1)	383.8 (275.9)
CD4 Percent	30.7 (79.2)	16.5(9.8)	27.1 (61.2)
Viral Load	3252.0 (2744.2)	203614.0 (427737.0)	43690.0 (92292.0)

Table 5 shows the relationship between HIV specific symptoms, common medical symptoms and indicators of disease severity summed across years. Disease severity was not significantly related to HIV specific symptom number. However, the relationship between common medical symptoms and CD4 count approached significance ($F(2,29) = 2.91, p < .07$).

Consultations and Procedures

Referrals for surgical or medical consultation and for diagnostic procedures (e.g., x-rays, etc.) and hospitalizations in the reporting period (between the last previous visit and the current visit) were recorded in specific data fields. Four patients were hospitalized a total of seven times, and seven patients were seen in an emergency room a total of 11 times. Conditions requiring use of emergency rooms (often triaged by the HOPES clinic nurse for appropriateness) included seizure control, injectable pain medications, and serious acute illness. Surgical referrals were infrequent with two patients referred for four procedures. Medical consultations were more frequently requested (10 patients for 16 consultations) and included referrals to dermatologists, neurologists, psychologists/psychiatrists, dentists and gastroenterologists. These referrals correlated with the number and diversity of medical conditions reported in the medical chart. In addition, eight patients were referred back to their primary care physicians a total of 51 times for management of routine non-HIV medical conditions.

Substance Use

Statistical relationships between alcohol problems, tobacco, illicit and injection drug use and the average number of medical symptoms per office visit, viral load, CD4 counts and CD4 percents were examined with one-way ANOVAs separately for each year (1995-1997). Tobacco, alcohol problems and drug use were not found to be related to either HIV specific conditions (weight loss > 10%, night sweats, diarrhea > 1 month, shingles, peripheral

TABLE 5. Number and Percent of CD4 Cells and Viral Load by Symptom Number

Measure (mean & standard deviation)	HIV Symptoms	
	Fewer than 5	5 or more
CD4 Count	237.0 (201.9)	165.2 (142.6)
CD4 Percent	14.0 (8.2)	10.5 (6.0)
Viral Load	42905 (100718)	*

	Common Medical Symptoms		
	Fewer than 5	5 to 14	15 or more
CD4 Count	410.1 (398.1)	304.7 (190.1)	136.9 (147.5)
CD4 Percent	69.6 (137.8)	19.1 (9.2)	10.0 (7.7)
Viral Load	19052 (40153)	6529 (5960)	92773 (154471)

Note. *Insufficient data.

neuropathy, mucosal candidiasis) or common health symptoms (fatigue, chronic pain, fever, nausea, upper respiratory infection, etc.). However, injection drug use was significantly related to reporting of specific HIV-related symptoms in 1995 [$F(1, 27) = 7.04$, $p < .05$], to commonly reported symptoms in 1996 [$F(1, 27) = 5.66$, $p < .05$] and to HIV specific symptoms for all three years combined [$F(1, 27) = 5.33$, $p < .05$].

The number of ICD-9 symptoms reported was about two times greater among patients reporting a history of alcohol problems and nearly three times greater among patients reporting a history of injection drug use. The alcohol relationship approached significance in 1995 and 1996 and was significant in 1997 [$F(2, 29) = 4.50$, $p < .05$]. The higher symptom reporting among those with a history of injection drug use was significant in 1996 [$F(1, 27) = 7.43$, $p < .05$] and 1997 [$F(1, 29) = 13.62$, $p < .001$].

CD4 absolute numbers, percentages and viral loads by substance use history are shown in Table 6. HIV status tended to be better in never users of tobacco, drugs, needles and those without alcohol problems, but none of these apparent differences were statistically significant.

TABLE 6. Number and Percent of CD4 Cells and Viral Load by Substance Abuse History

Measure (mean & standard deviation)	Substance Abuse History		
	Never	Past	Today
Alcohol Problems			
	(*n* = 15)	(*n* = 12)	*
CD4 Count	315.1(306.1)	266.9(208.5)	*
CD4 Percent	44.2(101.6)	14.4(9.0)	*
Viral Load	51775 (94186)	9531.7(4122)	*
´Cigarette Use			
	(*n* = 10)	(*n* = 6)	(*n* = 10)
CD4 Count	382.7(224.9)	184.5(154.1)	294.2(349.3)
CD4 Percent	55.5(124.3)	11.2(7.4)	19.5 (15.5)
Viral Load	15839 (17655)	*	73902(116721)
Drug Use			
	(*n* = 12)	(*n* = 11)	*
CD4 Count	316.6(343.5)	315.5(208.1)	*
CD4 Percent	16.2(15.0)	55.2(124.4)	*
Viral Load	58712 (99501)	7426(4668)	*
Injection Drug Use			
	(*n* = 21)	(*n* = 6)	*
CD4 Count	319.4(290.9)	205.3(165.6)	*
CD4 Percent	35.8(86.2)	13.0(9.3)	*
Viral Load	47405 (89073)	*	*

Note. *Insufficient data or not applicable.

DISCUSSION

The primary objective of this paper was to describe the medical status of patients in a community HIV clinic. The use of a computerized medical module proved to be key in developing the information in a format that could be evaluated. The medical module was designed with convenient entry options under an assumption that certain infections and health problems (those noted above) would be commonly encountered in the medical charts of HIV positive patients. The assumption of high rates of occurrence was borne out for many of the HIV-related symptoms and common health problems, but not for opportunistic infections or medical conditions. The medical problems that were commonly reported by patients at this clinic during this time period were largely of an acute, non-specific, non-emergent nature and included fatigue, headaches, night sweats and rash. HIV-related conditions of neuropathy (50%), pain (19%), and medication side effects (26.3%) were also commonly reported highlighting the dichotomous nature of HIV disease and the need for interventions from both primary care providers and HIV specialists to improve outcomes.

The data allowed us to examine whether the frequency of these symptoms and medical problems were greater in patients with poorer HIV status in terms of viral load and CD4 level. Analysis of the data over time demonstrated general improvement in the CD4 and viral load measurements that correlated with the increased use of protease inhibitors and combination therapy. However, even though this sample included patients with a wide range viral loads and CD4 counts, there were no significant correlations with the frequency of medical symptoms or conditions. One explanation is that severity of disease rather than number of symptoms is more sensitive to differences in these laboratory measures. Therefore, to provide a more complete medical record and to test this hypothesis it is recommended that severity ratings of symptoms/illnesses routinely be provided as part of the medical and nursing assessments.

The analysis also suggested that patients with a history of alcohol problems or injection drug use continue to have higher rates of medical symptom complaints of all types for years beyond the reported end of the substance problem, even though their HIV status in terms of CD4 counts or viral load was not found to differ from that of patients without a substance abuse history. An assessment of this history may give an important perspective in managing HIV treatment.

A secondary goal of this chart review and analysis was to assist with quality assurance review in the areas of consistency, completeness, follow-up, and documentation. Resulting recommendations included use of a rating of symptom severity to enhance completeness and documentation. The most useful part of the data entry module proved to be the non-specific fields available to enter ICD-9 codes for symptoms and diseases believed to be too infrequent to warrant a specific listing. Therefore, it is recommended that ICD-9 codes be used as the preferred method for building a database of symptoms/illnesses as they are particularly suitable for data compilation and analysis.

This review of HIV-positive patients' histories indicated several record keeping modifications that could lead to more consistent and descriptive information. All symptoms were entered in the database as being present only if recorded by either the doctor or the nurse at a patient visit. With visits used as the unit of measure, the concordance of reporting between doctors and nurses was examined. For the symptoms of diarrhea and night sweats, the consistency in reporting was 82.2% for diarrhea and 83.8% for night sweats. Most of the inconsistencies were due to these symptoms being reported by the nurse but not by the doctor at the same visit. Nurses recorded information during the patient visit on a form and the doctor dictated or wrote a clinic note after the visit without using a form. Diarrhea and night sweats were among the symptoms listed as specific options on the nurses' form.

Symptom reporting was usually non-specific and did not allow for quantification of severity. For example, documentation of frequency (e.g., "every day"), use of descriptive terms (e.g., "watery"), or discussion of cause (e.g., "with Norvir") or treatment efficacy (e.g., "resolved with Imodium") was found only occasionally. Symptom follow-up from one examination to the next was inconsistent, and it was difficult to discern whether the problem had in fact resolved. A follow-up system for symptoms (e.g., resolved, better, same, worse) would give the data more impact and be a clinical reminder to track earlier and persistent problems. In a similar vein, it is important to assess and to document medication adherence, not only for HIV specific agents, but also for others for which efficacy may differ depending on consistency of usage.

Nurses and physicians performed separate assessments at nearly all visits at this clinic and their consistency in reporting common patient symptoms was more than 80%. The most frequent source of inconsistencies was reporting of symptoms/illnesses by nursing staff but not by the physicians. It is recommended that the paper form used by nurses to check off symptoms and conditions found in their assessment also be reviewed by the physician at the same clinic visit to confirm the presence and character of each symptom or condition.

Another recommendation that our assessment of quality of care through chart review has suggested is that each symptom or illnesses be carried forward to the next clinic visit on the nurses' paper assessment form. This is a means to insure that each symptom or illnesses identified at the previous clinic visit is reassessed and that the follow-up is complete and documented. A method of categorizing symptom progress (e.g., resolved, better, same, worse) should be tested. If the symptom has changed (e.g., an infection becomes specified after lab results have been returned), perhaps a "changed" category, independent of the severity rating should be included.

In addition to suggesting modifications that may strengthen quality assurance, this database and analysis offers the possibility of exploring hypotheses specific to our nutrition project. Even in the absence of the suggested changes, some questions are accessible from the data in their present form. For example, is the number of symptoms statistically related to nutritional status? Does nutritional intervention impact the number of symptoms/illnesses? How does HIV drug therapy relate to the number and types of symptoms/illnesses and to nutritional status? A larger sample and more time points are probably necessary to provide a definitive answer to whether there is a relationship between laboratory measures of HIV status and number of illnesses/symptoms. All of these data have important implications for the practice of providing care to HIV-positive patients.

REFERENCES

Centers for Disease Control and Prevention. (1992). 1993 revised classification system for HIV infection and expanded surveillance case definition for AIDS among adolescents and adults. *Morbidity and Mortality Weekly Report, 41* (51), 961-62.

Scott, B. J., Larson, T. A., Brunner, R. L., Navarro, S., & Mathes, M. (1999). Evolution of nutrition screening services in a community based HIV clinic. *HIV Resource Review, 3* (6), 1-8.

Index

Page numbers followed by "t" indicate tables; page numbers followed by "f" indicate figures.

T - #0496 - 101024 - C0 - 212/152/16 - PB - 9780789011916 - Gloss Lamination